THE WHEEL OF YOU

A Guide to a Healthier, Happier, and Longer Life

Michael Doyle

ISBN-13: 9798873186754

Editor: Charmaine Smith

Cover design by: Michael Doyle
Printed in the United States of America

This book is not intended as a substitute for the medical advice of physicians or for psychiatric care.

CONTENTS

PREFACE

My intention in writing this book is to provide guidance and inspiration on how to live a healthier, happier, and longer life. However, there are no claims as to the effectiveness of this advice or any guarantees on results. Every individual must take responsibility for their own actions. Further research and reaffirmation of the advice contained within is not only expected but encouraged. Each person will have different results, and your own results will depend on how much time and effort you put into changing your life. New breakthroughs happen all the time and we are constantly increasing our knowledge and understanding of our bodies and the aging process. Keep learning, striving, and questioning every single day so you can be the best you can be and enjoy life to its fullest.

INTRODUCTION

If you are looking at this book, it is likely that you have already spent a lot of time looking for a way to live a longer, happier, and healthier life. You can take comfort that you are not alone in striving to achieve these goals. This quest is as old as humankind itself and almost universal but seems difficult to complete despite great advances in medicine and a plethora of information available across the internet. The overwhelming amount of data only confuses the issue. Every day there is more and more conflicting information. One day eggs are good for you and the next they are not. The same is true for wine, coffee, chocolate, and a whole host of other foods. It is almost impossible to know what or whom to listen to. This book is not intended to tell you what exactly to do, but to guide you in determining what advice to listen to and finding the best overall approach for you.

Each of the separate goals of health, longevity, and happiness is worthy of pursuing individually, but you might not realize that these goals are interdependent: Each component helps support the others. Imagine that you are a wheel with three spokes to support you as you travel through life. Each spoke must be sturdy and well maintained for the wheel to turn effectively. Any weak spoke will put undue stress on the other spokes, eventually causing the wheel to fail. This book will help you see how your mental, physical, and spiritual well-being interact and how developing each of these aspects of yourself contributes to your overall well-being.

Before we start down the road to becoming a more well-rounded individual, you must realize there is no shortcut. There is no shot, vitamin supplement, or magic workout that will cause you to achieve your goals. You will need determination, work, and patience. Taking care of your wheel needs to become a habit, not a whim or fad that you briefly pick up. As with any goal that is worth pursuing, you will have to overcome a wide variety of challenges. You can expect setbacks and periods where it seems you are not making any progress, but if you hang in there you will find the right combination of activities that works for you.

Unfortunately, there is no single series of steps that will guarantee results for everyone as some popular self-improvement systems suggest. For you to succeed you will have to change what you do daily. This process will take time and an extended effort for the rest of your life. You must build a system to maintain your wheel, re-evaluate it regularly, and adapt it over time so it can meet your unique needs at each time in your life. Variables such as your current progress, age, and life events will require you to evolve and adjust your system. As your challenges change, so will the way you approach them. Do not be too worried about the difficulties and changes you will have to face. The most important decision is when to start changing the way you spend the rest of your life.

Once you actually decide you want to make serious changes, you will start to see the results and improvements in how you look and feel. Of course, the amount of change that occurs will depend on how dedicated you are to making positive changes. It might sound as if you have to turn your life upside down, but that is far from the truth. Any step forward is a good step. No matter how small that step is, the most important thing is to just take that step and keep moving forward.

Of all the things you can do to improve your life, adjusting your attitude is the most important step and the one you have the most control over. It may sound like a cliché, but no matter what difficulties life throws at you, you always have the power to determine how you react to them.

You have probably heard the saying that if you give someone a fish you feed them for a day, but if you teach them to fish you have fed them for a lifetime. That is precisely my goal with this book. I do not want to give you a quick fix that will temporarily soothe your symptoms. I want to help you learn to develop habits and techniques for living a longer, healthier, and more fulfilling life for years to come without further help from me or anyone else. I am doing my part by writing this book and suggesting certain changes you can make, but you will have to do your part. Nobody can force you to change unless you really want to. You will have to use trial and error in finding out how to make life-altering changes that work for you. Your solution will be unique to you, and you will have to adjust it over time to accommodate changes in your body, mind, and spirit, such as the inevitable changes of aging.

First, we will try to find out what works for you in the present moment. We will come up with an initial plan and determine what to change when your current plan stops producing the results you want. There are many factors that will affect your plan, like genetics, environment, current age, past injuries, and situational stress factors. Hopefully your plan will give you a long and healthy life that lets you enjoy all the amazing things out there in this big wonderful world we inhabit.

Writing a book takes a huge amount of time and effort, and every author puts a part of themselves into the works they create. I truly hope that reading this book will help bring a positive change to the way you lead your life, as the writing of it has done for me. My wish is that the changes improve not only your life but also the lives of those around you and, in turn, the world in which we live. If that happens for just one other person, I have achieved my goal in writing this book and I will feel that it has truly been worth the effort.

CHAPTER 1: THE WHEEL OF YOU

What Is The Wheel Of You?

The Wheel of You is a wheel with various parts that make up who you are. The hub of the wheel is your inner self, and the rim of the wheel is the part you present to the world. Your wheel has three spokes—your physical, mental, and spiritual aspects—that support your rim as you travel through life. Just like a real wheel, each of your spokes needs to be strong to avoid burdening the other spokes and to support the rim equally. And you need a healthy, balanced rim that can handle life's weight without distorting.

The Wheel of You turns day after day, taking you on a hopefully long journey through life. A strong wheel makes the hills easier to climb, the bumps in the road less damaging, and the slopes more fun to speed down. Close your eyes and imagine yourself as this wheel. See how each spoke receives more stress at different times and has to be sturdy for the wheel to work properly. A single weak spoke shifts more stress to the other spokes and eventually weakens them and the entire wheel. For a truly balanced wheel, you must take care of each spoke with proper exercise and maintenance, or the whole Wheel of You suffers.

Why envision yourself as a wheel? What difference does it make how you see yourself within your mind and throughout the day? It matters because it helps you see how all the pieces fit together so you don't forget that you need to take care of your whole self, not just certain parts. Just as a flag might remind you of your country, images are powerful, and they can impact you in ways you are not consciously aware of.

Take the image of the Wheel and hold it in your mind to keep you vigilant in your quest for a better you. Think about how each activity you do to improve yourself affects your wheel. Think about whether you are neglecting any of your spokes. Doing this will also help you incorporate other aspects of the wheel into your day-to-day activities. Later in the book we will talk about various activities and how they can be modified to enhance all of your spokes.

The Physical Spoke

This is the easiest spoke for most of us to comprehend because it is the most visually accessible. It only takes a moment to look at the scale and see how much weight you have gained or lost during the week or to see how your body looks in the mirror. Anybody can determine how many pounds they can bench-press or how many miles they can run in a certain amount of time. These are numbers, and we are used to numbers. They make us feel comfortable (or uncomfortable as the case may be). That is why many people focus on this spoke to the detriment of the others. Focusing on the physical spoke and making it stronger is not a bad thing, but the effort you put in needs to be balanced with the other aspects of the wheel so it does not weaken and start to fail.

The mental and spiritual spokes are just as important as the physical but are less easily measured and may be neglected for this reason. Fortunately, a lot of the activities that strengthen the physical spoke can also benefit the mental and spiritual spokes. For example, walking requires considerable brain processing power you are probably unaware of consciously. This is especially true if you vary the path where you walk so you have to make decisions on where to head and take in the sights around you.

A walk in nature can definitely benefit your spiritual spoke, and because your foot must adjust to the varying terrain, your mind gets a workout as well.

There is more to the physical spoke than just the obvious things we can measure (pounds lifted, reps done, miles walked, etc.). Watch a small child as they are learning how to walk. You can see how much thought it takes to move that foot forward and put it down in a place that will keep them from falling over. There are literally thousands of neurons being fired with every step you take. As you get older your brain compartmentalizes the process of walking so your conscious mind can focus on higher-functioning tasks. As long as you keep performing a routine activity (walking in this case), your brain can take care of that task in the background. But if you neglect that activity those pathways will start to deteriorate, making it harder to perform that function in the future.

The Mental Spoke

In the past the brain was seen as static once you grow to adulthood and then declining as you age, with no other options. While I was growing up, most of the information out there said brain cells die and are never replaced, that our brains were destined to constantly atrophy and that nothing we could do would prevent it. The only thing we could change was the rate of shrinkage. Recent research has shown that idea to be untrue. Our brains can replace lost cells and repair damage if we treat them well and train them. As further research is released, I believe we will learn that the brain behaves much like a muscle that needs to be exercised to maintain its size, shape, and flexibility.

A healthy mind is key to enjoying life and cannot be neglected, especially if you want to enjoy your later years. In this book we will discuss ways to exercise your mind and keep it youthful. No matter what your age, there are activities you can do to stimulate your mind. Don't worry, you do not have to be born a genius or study all the time. You just have to exercise your mind. But the mind is complex, with a wide array of different components that need individual attention. Just like your muscles, all of these functions of the brain (language, math, music, reading, physical and emotional functioning, etc.) need exercise to stay in shape.

Despite our best efforts, events happen in our lives that can impair our mental faculties. A variety of diseases and injuries can impact the strength of your mental spoke, but if you start off with the goal of a well-balanced mental state and a healthy wheel overall, you can minimize the effects of these unforeseen life events. We now know the brain is remarkably resilient, even shifting duties from one part of the brain to the other when necessary. Even people who have suffered severe head trauma have been able to live normal lives. The best thing you can do for your brain's health is to keep it active, exposing it to new and challenging information so it is ready to take on life's challenges.

An active mind is your brain's best defense, better than any drugs or herbs you might take. Not to say these supplements have no benefits, but you won't get stronger just by losing weight and not doing any exercise. Your muscles become weak and flabby without use no matter what steroids or supplements you take. So get out there and try new things, visit new places, and learn new skills if you want to keep your brain in good shape at any age.

The Spiritual Spoke

This spoke is the most difficult one to quantify. Society has spent a lot of time developing measurements for mental and physical attributes, but very few to determine how well your spiritual self is doing. Without a doubt, it is difficult to determine the strength of this spoke. Many people think they are doing well spiritually until some unexpected stress factor arrives. Spiritual strength runs deep and true. It will carry you through the most difficult times and keep you humble during the best times. No matter what religion you are or whether you are atheist or agnostic, your spiritual strength is every bit as important as your physical and mental strength. Just like your other spokes, the spiritual spoke requires regular upkeep. It is not simply present or absent. Like physical exercise, this maintenance comes easier for some people than others, but you can do it if you make it a priority and are willing to put in the effort.

If you do nothing else for your spiritual self, then do this one thing: Believe in yourself. If you don't, how can you expect anyone else to believe in you? This is truly an arduous task for many people. Even those who seem self-assured may harbor extreme levels of self-doubt and loathing. To get past those feelings you will have to find your own self-worth and not depend on the validation of others. If you are happy with yourself, it matters little what others think.

The Core Of The Wheel

After stripping away all your personal perceptions, how other people view you, and the defenses the subconscious puts up to protect you, we can finally get to your core. The core is who you truly are deep down. Don't worry, this is not going to devolve into a religious sermon, but in order to make yourself a better person you need to figure out who you truly are. It is important to realize that you do have an inner self and it needs to be protected from damage.

As long as your spokes (mental, physical, and spiritual) are in good shape, they protect your core and minimize damage to it. It is much easier to repair damage to one of your spokes than to your core. Such damage usually occurs around significant life events such as the death of someone close to you or the severing of a long-term relationship. At times, damage to your core will be almost impossible to repair and will make your wheel more susceptible to further damage. Therefore, it is important to keep your spokes as strong as possible to protect your core and help you rebound from life's inevitable stressful events.

The Rim Of The Wheel

You can think of the rim as the part of you that is exposed to the world and to all the trials and tribulations of everyday life. Your rim is the part of you that you let others see and controls how they see you. Your travel through life weathers it and assaults it daily.

The rim has two primary purposes: to give you a surface to roll through life on and a framework to protect your core. Just like the rim of a real wheel, it needs sturdy spokes for support. A weakness in any spoke can expose the core to damage and weaken the other spokes.

It may help to envision yourself riding through life on the rim of your wheel just as with riding a bike or driving a car. If you were riding a bike and saw a bunch of broken glass, you would try to avoid it to save your tires and avoid crashing. If you can easily avoid damage to your wheel, you should. This might sound like common sense, but people constantly put themselves in harm's way. This goes for anything unnecessary you apply to your body, whether drugs, needles, or physical damage. When your wheel is young and strong you can take a lot of damage, but that damage can add up and become permanent, affecting your wheel for the rest of your journey. Just keep the image of your wheel in mind when deciding what actions to take. Think about the long-term effects of your choices. We have all made decisions that have damaged the strength of our wheel, but we can all learn from these lessons and do what we can to protect our wheel for a long and healthy future.

The Quick Fix

This book is not about the quick fix. The pursuit of so-called quick fixes is almost always detrimental to your long-term health. Unfortunately, we have become a society fixated on those kinds of results. We are bombarded daily with "facts" that are simply designed to grab our attention and ultimately grab the money from our wallet. Hopefully you want health and happiness for the long term. Making permanent day-to-day lifestyle changes will best help you achieve this goal. Creating and maintaining your wheel requires daily diligence and a focus on long-term results.

As an example of a popular quick fix, let us take a look at performance-enhancing steroids. These steroids can help improve your physical spoke in the short term. You will gain muscle mass quickly and will start to look stronger provided you exercise while you take them. The results will usually be visible quickly, which encourages you to take more steroids. It sounds great in the short term, but the problem is with the steroids' long-term effects. Steroid abuse can lead to a whole host of problems, including fits of rage, deterioration of your joints, unwanted hair, baldness, and even premature death. Regular workouts and a good diet will provide most people with a firm, physically fit body they can be proud of without the need for steroids. It will take longer, but the results will last longer and you are more likely to establish the healthy habits needed for a more satisfying life in your later years.

My final quick-fix advice is not to rely on gadgets, crazy diets, or fad workout regimens unless you are going to incorporate them into your regular routine. Most of these quick-fix gimmicks leave the person back where they started or even worse off. For one thing, these gimmicks usually focus on one spoke and not the whole wheel. To be truly successful, any plan to make a better you has to incorporate all three spokes. Second, most gimmicks are designed to make money for those who promote them, who will do whatever they can to make as much as they can from you in the shortest time possible. There is no profit for them if their advice actually works in the long term. They would lose repeat business if it did.

I am not trying to say there is no benefit from some of the solutions out there but that you should approach them as components of a much larger plan if you hope to have any kind of success. Always approach these solutions with a critical eye, for there are definitely programs that do more harm than good. It is wise in my opinion to rely on programs that have stood the test of time rather than one of the countless get-fit-quick scams that are ever present.

CHAPTER 2: PHYSICAL SPOKE BASICS

Genetics

Let's get the bad news out of the way. You are pretty much stuck with the genes your mom and dad gave you, at least for the time being. In the not too distant future, gene therapy will be available to alter some things you might want to change, like curing baldness or making you store fat less easily. Sounds like science fiction, but we really aren't that far away. In the meantime you need to work with what your parents gave you. Some of us may never be able to dunk a basketball or bench-press 300 pounds. You may be stuck with premature baldness or even be unlucky enough to have a rare genetic disease. These things you can't change, at least for now, so focus on what you can do with what you have. This will help you physically as well as spiritually.

The good news is that once you identify the items you need to focus on, you can develop a physical regimen that is designed just for you. If you have a genetic tendency to store fat more easily, you will need to focus on activities that burn calories and other ways to increase your metabolism, and focus on how many calories you consume. The truth is that everybody's genetic makeup (except identical twins and triplets of course) is different and the needs of each body are equally unique. It will take some effort to decide on your goals and identify the activities you need in order to meet them. We will discuss some exercises and activities later in this book that will let you focus on specific areas and provide a balanced approach so you can do your best to take care of your physical spoke for many, many years to come.

Your Maintenance Plan

It is a common belief that some physical things, like balance, eyesight, and bone density, just get worse as you get older and there is not much you can do about it. This is still currently true for a lot of the physical parts of aging, but you can slow down or even reverse many aging processes. You can think of your body as a car that has to be maintained. A car well cared for can run for hundreds of thousands of miles and still look great. You can do the same thing for your body by taking care of yourself. Later in this book we will work on developing an overall maintenance plan that will help you minimize the physical effects of aging.

Balance

Maintaining your ability to balance is essential to enjoying your later years. A lot of people will tell you that your balance will only get worse as you get older. It may be true that your maximum ability to balance decreases slowly as you get older, but few people achieve that level of balancing ability. For example, I have better balance now than I did in my twenties. Several years ago I would never have been able to maintain a dancing warrior pose, but I can do it easily now. This is because balance uses core muscles that most of us do not normally exercise in our day-to-day activities. For example, sitting at a desk all day does not help improve your balance.

Balance needs practice to be maintained. I find that yoga is the best way for me to maintain and improve my balance, but there are other ways to maintain this aspect of the physical spoke. A variety of exercises have been developed that concentrate on your core muscles and therefore improve your balance. The main reason balance is so important is that it keeps you from falling over and possibly injuring yourself in your later years. Well-developed balance will help prevent you from breaking a hip or leg. Balance is a cooperation between your muscles and brain that keeps you in tune with your surroundings. Maintaining your balance will help protect both your mental and physical well-being. Avoiding physical damage from a fall will also help maintain your whole wheel. I have seen many people deteriorate in all their spokes after a fall that breaks a hip or leg. It is a domino effect that can cause depression, bone loss, and mental degradation. All of this stemmed from a simple fall they could have avoided by properly maintaining their balance.

Bone Density

Your bones are not just stone sticks that exist in your body and slowly wear away over time. They are living components in constant flux. They change in density depending on how they are used. Proper blood flow and nutrients are also required for bones to be healthy.

Bones do far more than support the rest of your body. Some bones such as femurs produce the blood cells your body needs. Much like muscles or your brain, bones need to be "exercised" to maintain their optimum strength and performance. This is done by giving them the proper nutrients and putting the proper amounts of pressure on them.

The weight of your body puts a certain amount of pressure on your bones. For example, just standing around will cause gravity to exert pressure on the bones of your legs, hips, and spine. This causes your body to react and keep a certain level of calcium in your bones, keeping them strong and functional. In outer space there is no gravity, so your bones start to lose density. Astronauts try to compensate by doing exercises that put pressure on their bones. Otherwise, long-term astronauts' bones would become weak and unable to support their weight when they come back to earth.

Lifting weights is a great way to help maintain your bone

density. This can be done in the traditional way with free weights, using resistance machines, or even doing something basic like push-ups. The increased pressure on your bones signals your body to strengthen them. Your body does not want to waste energy and materials on maintaining parts of your body that are not being used. This principle holds true for most of the parts of your body and brain. If you don't like lifting free weights, there are many ways to help increase your bone density, such as hiking with a backpack. The additional weight of the backpack increases the pressure on your bones and joints, much like being in a higher-gravity environment. Hiking regularly will make your bones stronger over time.

Eyes

Eyesight is something everyone can improve and maintain but most people ignore. We use crutches such as eyeglasses and contact lenses to help us see instead of strengthening our eyes through exercise. I am not suggesting you can fix everything that is wrong with your eyes through exercises, but you can keep them from getting weaker. As a child, I had to wear glasses from the age of seven. I wore them for well over twenty years before I started exercising my eyes daily, and after a few years I was able to pass my eye exam with ease. Mostly I focused on items that were close and then on items far away. I would repeat this over and over on my walks. I also made a point of not staring at my computer screen for too long. I would take frequent breaks to rest my eyes. There are various books available that can give you more details, but the simple steps mentioned above give me significant results. A proper diet containing the vitamins the eyes need, such as vitamin A, is also essential for eye health.

It is often said that the eyes are the gateway to the soul. To some extent that is true, since your emotions and your health are reflected in your eyes. If you are not physically well, your eyes may have dark circles under them or may be discolored. Dark circles can be caused by many factors such as allergies, lack of sleep, stress, eye strain, and other ailments. If you constantly see dark circles under your eyes, you should try to figure out the cause and take steps to remedy it.

On a personal note, for a long time I often felt tired during the day and saw dark circles under my eyes but could not identify the cause. It turned out that I have a severe allergy to mold. The causes were my basement, compost bin, and the dead leaves in my yard. Regardless of how much sleep I got, I still felt and looked tired. I was using a lot of antihistamines to try to control the symptoms, but now I control them by removing the sources of the mold and therefore have a lot more energy. The dark circles are starting to disappear, and I feel much more alert and energetic. It is worth your effort to identify the source of your allergies if you have them and figure out how to minimize your exposure.

Hair And Nails

The health of your hair is also an important indicator of your overall health. A good diet and exercise can help to improve your hair, but you are also at the mercy of genetics here, especially if you have premature gray hair or are going bald. I have had gray hair since I was in my early twenties, and other than dyeing my hair there was not much I could do. With advances in science, you can reverse some of the effects of premature graying, but gray hair is just a fact of life for now. If it really bothers you then go ahead and dye it, but gray hair by itself does not mean much in terms of your health. The sheen of your hair is a far more important indicator. If you are healthy, your hair should have a nice healthy sheen to it. If you are not healthy, it is likely that your hair will appear dull and lifeless no matter what products you use.

Balding is primarily driven by genetics, but there can be other contributors such as stress. Science has made significant gains with baldness, but it still plagues many people, mainly men, but some women too. Baldness can greatly affect your self-esteem, and if it really bothers you, you should take steps to remedy or minimize it. Just telling yourself to embrace being bald is generally not very helpful. You should do what you need to do to feel good about how you look. My only advice here is to be careful about what products you choose and do your research before spending a lot of money on a remedy that may not work.

Your nails are another indicator of your health and diet. If they are yellow or brittle, it means that your diet is lacking and/or your health is poor. It could mean something simple, like not making or eating enough collagen, or it could indicate something far more serious. If you notice your nails look unhealthy, you should consult a doctor to identify the cause. Besides being yellow or brittle, nails can be affected by a fungus which causes odor and discoloration but is easily treated. Whatever the cause of your unhealthy-looking nails, it should be addressed and monitored so you can be healthy overall and feel good about yourself and how others see you.

Flexibility

Maintaining your flexibility may not sound important to having a long, healthy life, but it becomes increasingly significant as we age. It can help keep you from spraining a muscle, tearing a ligament, or even breaking a hip. It also keeps your body from getting stiff and decaying. Just as a car has to be lubed to perform well, flexibility has to be maintained and worked on regularly. For most people, flexibility will decrease as you get older unless you take steps to counter this.

Without doing something to counteract the negative effects of aging in your routine, the tendons and joints will become dry and brittle, making them more likely to be damaged. Luckily, with some effort you can maintain flexibility throughout your lifetime. There are many people in advanced years who have great flexibility. I have seen people in their nineties who are more flexible than many in their twenties. Personally, I am far more flexible now than I was in my early twenties and thirties and continue to get more flexible as I work on it steadily.

Practicing yoga on a regular basis is one of the best ways I have found to maintain flexibility. If your schedule doesn't allow for taking regular classes or you just don't enjoy it, you could try attending an occasional yoga class just to help you maintain your flexibility. Of course, any kind of exercise where you are moving your body parts more than you normally do will help maintain your flexibility, but I find that yoga pushes me to increase my flexibility in a way I haven't encountered in any other exercise. Many types of martial arts also focus on flexibility and are adequate alternatives. If you enjoy neither yoga nor martial arts, you should at least stretch on a regular basis. Your body will thank you for it.

An additional benefit of working on your flexibility is that it helps move fluid through your lymphatic system. This will help you to fight off diseases and may even prevent a whole host of autoimmune illnesses. Studies are needed to determine just how effective increased flexibility is in protecting you from getting sick, but there is no doubt it is key to having a more enjoyable later life.

Joints

The joints in your body are essential for you to move through life. They are also some of the most easily damaged parts of your body and are very hard to heal. Much like the moving parts in a car, they require lubrication. Instead of oil, your body uses a substance called synovial fluid. Without synovial fluid your joints grind together, creating friction and causing wear and tear that is hard for your body to overcome. Your body can repair small amounts of damage without outside help, but more significant damage requires medical attention. Severe damage may even require surgery. Despite advances in modern medicine, there is nothing that can totally replace synovial fluid.

If you are unfortunate enough to seriously damage one of your joints, as most of us will do in our lifetimes, it is important that you don't try to fully use those joints too soon. You will feel completely healed long before your joints are ready to be fully used. Until joints are almost one hundred percent back to normal, they can easily be re-damaged. Also, the muscles surrounding the joint will be weakened after the injury and less able to support the area around the joint until they return to normal strength. Physical therapy can help restore this strength, but until you can start regularly using the joint again, you will have to increase the pressure on it in stages.

Certain activities like basketball, soccer, and hockey are riskier for causing joint injuries. While these are great physical activities and can provide many benefits for the entire wheel, almost everyone I know who has played them as an adult has suffered joint injuries. If you choose to participate in these sports, you need to take special care of your joints. This might mean putting your ego aside rather than pushing yourself too far. Making that awesome catch or blocking a particularly difficult goal is not worth months of trying to heal yourself and a lifetime of nagging joint injury.

Kidneys

The kidneys are the purification filters of your body. Most toxins you put into your system pass through the kidneys, and they do their best to remove what they can. They take out these unwanted particles and send them out through your urine along with any excess water. While kidneys are essential to your well-being, you are blessed to have two of them though you only need one to survive. They are also one of the easier organs to transplant if you can find a suitable donor. Please do not go out and damage them, though. The risk and cost far outweigh any perceived benefit. You should do your best to take care of them so that they can function at the highest capacity to remove the toxic substances from your body.

Protein-focused diets are a popular way to lose weight, but if you eat a diet heavy in protein, your body has to excrete a lot of urea, putting a heavy load on your kidneys. This stresses your kidneys and if they can't process the extra urea, your body will start to suffer and eventually stop functioning. You could also develop kidney stones. A similar caution applies for many other substances we put into our bodies. Although some of them are harder on the kidneys than others, you should try to minimize any stressors. The most important principle here is to only consume the nutrients your body needs—to refrain from eating more protein than you need, taking more vitamins than you need, or consuming more medicine than you need. Follow this advice and both you and your kidneys will be thankful.

Kidneys function by processing fluid and therefore need fluid to function correctly. You can take care of your kidneys by making sure that you drink enough water throughout the day. Whether you hydrate with pure water or some other drink does not really matter unless it contains too many particles. Clean, relatively particle-free water is great, but if you consume your fluids in other ways such as tea or soda, you are still getting water into your body.

A lot of people think they need to consume "sports" drinks or liquids that are at the same particle level that your body supposedly should be. Unless you are exercising at a very high level and sweating copiously, you are perfectly fine never consuming these drinks. Your normal diet should give you adequate amounts of electrolytes. For example, a lot of these drinks contain potassium, which your body needs, but once you consume enough of it, the rest gets passed out of your body through your urine. In other words, when exercising, stick with water to quench your thirst and save some money and your kidneys' effort.

Liver

You probably never think about your liver until something goes wrong, despite it being one of the most important organs in your body. You simply cannot live without a liver. It is also the only organ that can regrow itself through regeneration. You can even cut off part of the liver and it will grow back. You can survive with a partial liver, even as little as 25%. A damaged liver can in some cases grow back to its normal size within a few weeks. This doesn't mean that you should abuse it, though. You should maintain it along with your other organs.

Your liver aids digestion by creating bile, but it is also responsible for detoxifying your bloodstream. Most people know of its ability to process alcohol and other toxins. It can easily process small amounts of alcohol, but large amounts of alcohol on a regular basis can cause severe liver damage. The exact number of functions the liver provides is still debated, but we know it is responsible for around 500 functions. By now it should be obvious that a healthy liver is key to having a long, healthy life. You can take care of your liver by not dumping too many toxins into it at once.

Moderation is the key to a healthy liver. This means eating a sensible diet and not putting too many non-food items into it such as excessive alcohol. Excess vitamins and minerals can also abnormally burden your liver (as well as your kidneys) because it will try to process these chemicals to the point of overload. Keeping your weight at a reasonable level is another important way to maintain your liver. When surrounded by fat, it becomes far less efficient.

Lungs

You may think there is not much you need to do to take care of your lungs. You just sit around and breathe and that's pretty much it. Of course, you probably know that smoking cigarettes is bad for your lungs. It would be hard to miss that information from the slew of media ads over the last few decades and the ban of smoking in many places. That prevention method is straightforward. Simply avoiding smoking is not enough, though. You need to be proactive in taking care of your lungs. They transfer life-giving oxygen into your bloodstream and remove carbon dioxide from your system. When they are impaired the rest of your body cannot function properly.

The first step in maintaining your lungs is to exercise them. There are two main points to consider when exercising your lungs. The first point is their elasticity. You want your lung tissues to be stretched out on a regular basis, much like your muscles. You can accomplish this by simply breathing in very deeply on a regular basis. This happens naturally if you are exercising, but you can do it even if you are not exercising by practicing deep breathing. Simply take in very deep breaths, hold for several seconds, then try to expel as much of the air as you can when you breathe out. This practice will also reduce stress and regulate your blood pressure. This doesn't sound difficult but is easy to forget. Deep breaths will also bring additional oxygen into the brain and make you more alert.

The second consideration when exercising your lungs is the dead space that exists within them. You can never empty your lungs completely, so there is always some dead space in which oxygen is transferred less efficiently. You just need to try to clean out the space in your lungs the best you can. The deep breathing exercises mentioned earlier and aerobic exercise will help to minimize the dead air space in your lungs.

In maintaining your lungs, it's also important to keep unwanted particles out of them. Almost everywhere we go there are damaging particles hovering around in the air. These particles can clog up the lungs and interfere with taking in oxygen. They can also cause allergic reactions, and some can even increase your chances of getting cancer. Our bodies are built to handle a certain level of these particulates, but heavy concentrations are not good for you even if naturally occurring, such as grass or tree pollen. During times of high concentrations of these particles you should try to be inside where you can filter the particles out of the air using filter systems. Another defense is to be near areas of running water like a river or the ocean.

If you must live in an area where the air quality is not good, you should try to do even more deep breathing and aerobic exercise (indoors in a filtered environment if possible) to help flush out these particles and keep your lungs in top condition. If you can, you should spend some time in areas with high-quality air such as near the ocean, where the particles have had a chance to be removed by falling to the water. Right after a rain or snowfall is good too. Take deep long breaths and hold them as long as comfortable, allowing the pure air to circulate inside you, then expel the bad air out into atmosphere.

Skin

Your skin is your first line of defense against a host of germs and viruses, radiation, the sun, physical damage, and anything else the world throws your way. Taking care of your skin is about more than trying to look good. If you take care of your skin, it will take care of you. The opposite is also true. Unhealthy skin can lead to infections, cuts, lesions, poor circulation, nutrient loss, and even cancer. Luckily, taking care of your skin isn't too complicated. The basics to taking care of your skin are as follows.

- Avoid damaging UV rays from the sun and/or tanning booths by using sunscreen and avoiding the sun around noon
- Keep your face clean daily
- Moisturize your skin even if it is oily
- Watch for any sudden changes in your skin such as rashes, sudden mole growth, or discoloration and see a doctor if these occur
- Eat a well-balanced diet

This advice applies to men just as much as women. Like most maintenance tasks, the sooner you start taking care of your skin, the better off you will be later in life. However, this is especially true for your skin. You can always potentially lose weight or fix your teeth, but skin damage is hard to repair and can have long-lasting effects that may not show up for years. Additionally, although some damage can be repaired, skin damage tends to be cumulative and may eventually require medical intervention to correct.

The skin is not an environment-proof barrier. It is porous and can absorb many different types of substances, such as steroids and nicotine. In fact, it is the preferred delivery system for drugs that might be hard on your liver because they can enter your blood system directly via the skin, bypassing the digestive system oral medication has to pass through. You should remember this fact when dealing with toxic substances such as cleansers and pesticides. If you do get a toxic chemical on you, the first thing you should do is wash the affected area with lots of water. Even if you are not sure about the substance, it is safer to go ahead and thoroughly clean the affected area.

Sleep

A decent night's sleep is essential to your mental, physical, and spiritual well-being. Getting a proper amount of sleep every night can be a challenge. Life happens and it is usually sleep that suffers first. Going to bed and getting up around the same time every day is ideal for optimizing our sleep, but the reality is most of us have hectic schedules and we end up getting off our routine. Just try and set a schedule and do your best to stick to it.

The quality of sleep is just as important as its length. You can sleep a full eight hours and still wake up tired if you are tossing and turning all night. These are some steps I take to help me get more restful slumber.

- Keep it dark. Even a small amount of light can cause disruption in sleep.
- Invest in a bed that is right for you. Most people spend a third of their life in bed, so it is worth it.
- Use a white noise generator or a fan to minimize noise disruptions.
- Keep the temperature set at a comfortable level and try not to sleep too close to a vent to keep the fluctuations to a minimum.
- Do something peaceful, like light reading, before you

fall asleep to help clear your mind.
- Avoid sugar and caffeine for at least a few hours before bed.
- Stay away from emitters of blue light like the television and phone an hour before trying to fall asleep.

The inability to sleep (chronic insomnia) is a serious matter and should be dealt with immediately. While it is true that lack of sleep can cause death (nobody has gone a full year sleepless without dying), that is rare. Of greater concern to most people is fitful and intermittent sleep that can affect your overall health. The times I have had trouble sleeping were stressful times in my life and luckily did not last too long. During stressful times, exercising a few hours before bed has helped tire my body out and let me get deep sleep. It does not always work, but it does help. The best solution is to try to alleviate the stress from your life, which will help you all around.

There are many medications out there that people use to help them sleep. I am not a big proponent of these medications because of their potential side effects and the danger of becoming reliant upon them. Too often, we try to medicate our way out of problems, and it ends up causing us more harm in the long run. However, medication may be necessary for some people, and if you truly do have serious sleeping issues it may be the right thing for you, but I would try other methods first. Several less drastic herbal remedies are available, like chamomile tea. Even a glass of wine before bed would be preferable to many of the over-the-counter and prescription medications available.

Thanks to recent advances in technology, the average person can now purchase wristbands that monitor your sleep patterns. There are several brands out there and the list keeps growing. These are generally designed to measure how deeply you sleep and for how long. The type of sleep that seems to be the most important is REM (rapid eye movement) sleep. This is when you typically dream, and your eyes will move rapidly. The longer the periods of REM, the deeper your sleep will be. While these devices do not make you sleep more deeply, they can help you monitor whether your sleep is getting more fitful so you can address that.

Teeth

Taking care of your teeth is one of the most important things you can do for yourself. With proper care, there is no reason that most people can't have healthy teeth their entire life. Having bad teeth can greatly affect all three of your spokes. It can affect your self-esteem, your appearance, and your ability to fight off diseases and can be a source of intense pain. Your genetics and early dental habits play a large part in the health of your teeth, but it is never too late to start taking care of your teeth. The straightforward steps to doing so are listed below.

- Floss on a regular basis
- Brush with fluoride every morning and night (and after eating a lot of sugar)
- Go the dentist twice a year

If those three steps are all you do, you have done most of the required maintenance and can hopefully enjoy a healthy smile for all your days.

Teeth are one of the few parts of the whole you that I fully support altering so that you can feel better about yourself. This could mean getting braces (even at an advanced age), having them whitened, or replacing them with artificial ones if they are damaged or need to be pulled. It is built into us to see someone with good looking teeth as healthy and practicing good hygiene. The best part of having healthy, good-looking teeth is that it helps you smile more, which is always a good thing.

The Food We Eat

We are all familiar (or should be) with the concept of calories. Calories are the fuel that powers us through the day. Almost every day we see signs about how many calories certain types of foods contain. I do not personally count calories, but it can be an effective method for those people who are trying to lose weight. This book is not designed to tell you how much or what to eat but to give you information so you can make those decisions for yourself based upon your goals for your body. Everyone's body is different and has different caloric requirements and may need different types of food. For example, some people are allergic or sensitive to certain foods and must replace them with alternatives. So, let's start with some basics about calories and then move onto some advanced subjects.

Fuel And Building Blocks

The human body is a machine that needs fuel as well as building materials. This is accomplished by processing the foods you consume. I put the foods we eat into two categories: fuel to propel us through our daily activities, and building materials for growing and repairing the body. Fuel is basically anything you ingest that your body can digest. This fuel usually falls into one of three categories: carbohydrates, fats, and proteins. All of these can be turned into fuel for the body. The most basic type of fuel is glucose, which can be used throughout the body to run it, just as your car uses gasoline.

The building blocks of your body are mostly made up of protein. You can convert protein into "fuel," but you cannot convert carbohydrates or fats into proteins since proteins contain nitrogen. Carbohydrates and fats are made of carbon, hydrogen, and oxygen. Therefore, you must consume protein to get the necessary building blocks to build or repair your body. It is important for us to look at each of these categories individually to better understand what they do for you. But in general, you need to vary your diet, consuming all three groups in the right proportions for your body's unique needs.

The number of calories you consume should match the number you use during the day to avoid gaining weight. For this purpose the total number of calories is more important than the type. For example, you can eat nothing but fat and still lose weight. This goes for any other type of calories you consume (including proteins and alcohol) if you burn up the calories you consume within a timely manner. If you eat a lot during the normal work week and then try to lose all those calories on the weekend you will burn fat, but you may burn up muscle as well. This is why you will see a lot of long-distance runners that look anorexic even though they are constantly working out. They are basically eating their muscles up faster than they create them through exercise.

The same thing goes for how much you eat at a time. If you only eat once a day, as sumo wrestlers do, your body must store those calories so you can fuel yourself through the rest of the day. Think of a car with a tank that stores fat as its gas. Cars that must go very long distances between fill-ups have to store a lot of gas. This means you should eat smaller meals throughout the day (unless you are training to be a sumo wrestler) so your body knows it has calories coming in and can safely use up its current reserves.

Besides fuel, your body needs to consume other things on a regular basis. Vitamins, minerals, fiber, and water are all necessary. Each of these components is important and deserves consideration. But first we are going to go over how much energy each type of food provides. The main categories are shown below.

Types Of Calories

- Carbohydrates – 4 calories per gram
- Protein – 4 calories per gram
- Fat – 9 calories per gram
- Alcohol – 7 calories per gram

Carbohydrates, fats, and alcohol are basically all broken down into simple sugars that are then used as energy or, in the case of excess calories, stored as fat. Proteins are used as protein if your body needs protein, but the excess is converted into sugars, releasing the nitrogen into your body which then gets released into your urine.

Your body has two main buckets, or ways to store calories. It stores them as simple sugars (i.e., glucose) in the blood for quick consumption and as fat for longer-term storage. (There is also the energy stored within cells in the form of ATP, but that is not important for this discussion.)

The blood sugar bucket empties quickly and needs to be low or empty before the fat bucket starts emptying. This is a simplification of the process, but it's good to keep in mind when you are deciding what to eat and how to lose weight if that is one of your goals. Quite a few variables can affect this equation such as the amounts of certain hormones (especially cortisol, estrogen, and testosterone) in your system, how quickly your body breaks down various types of calories, and how you burn calories (aerobically or anaerobically). Regardless of these variables, if you burn more calories than you consume you will lose weight, just as you will most likely gain weight if the opposite is true. The goal is to achieve a balance that works for you and not to have your weight fluctuate wildly up and down.

Carbohydrates

Carbohydrates (or carbs) are the basic fuel on which your body runs. A gram of carbohydrates is equal to 4 calories (actually kilocalories, but we usually just say calories) per gram, but all calories are not created equal. Some carbs are immediately usable by the body, while others must be broken down before the body can turn them into energy.

Carbohydrates are often referred to as sugars or starches and come in a wide variety of types. Despite this variety, carbs can be grouped into two basic categories. The first type is simple carbohydrates. These are also called simple sugars and can be used directly or broken down quickly to power your muscles and your brain as well as other functions of your body. The second type is complex carbohydrates. Complex carbohydrates take much longer to break down and can therefore provide energy for extended periods of time. The different types of simple carbohydrates are listed below.

Simple Carbohydrates

- Glucose
- Fructose
- Sucrose
- Galactose
- Lactose
- Dextrose

As mentioned earlier, simple carbohydrates can be directly absorbed into your bloodstream and are therefore available for immediate conversion into energy. This is very useful if you are doing activities that consume a lot of calories such as running or rigorous hiking. Ideally, you consume these simple carbohydrates either right before or during the activities so that you can use them right away. The reason that you want to consume them within a short amount of time is that your body can only keep a certain amount of them stored in the bloodstream. When your body has excess amounts of these sugars, they are converted into fat molecules and deposited in adipose tissue (fat cells) for future use.

Sources of Simple Carbohydrates

- Fruits
- Honey
- Beets
- Carrots
- Maltose
- Molasses
- Sweet corn
- Sweet onions
- Milk products

- Sugar cane

Raw fruits generally taste sweeter than cooked or processed fruits, and therefore less of them is required to satisfy your sweetness cravings. This is because fructose comes in multiple types but when heated up it turns into the less sweet forms of sugar. The sweeter version of fructose tastes almost twice as sweet as regular cane sugar, but the other version of fructose has about the same sweetness.

There are few foods that I am totally against, but high fructose corn syrup (HFCS) is one of them. Although it is simply a combination of fructose and glucose, it does not seem to sate your hunger like other sugars do. In other words, after eating foods sweetened with HFCS, you are still hungry. This sweetener is used for a lot of reasons, but cost is the main one. It is cheaply made in vast quantities from corn, and it stores for long periods of time without spoiling. The research is still out about the negative effects of HFCS on the human body, but many studies point to adverse health problems related to obesity tied to HFCS. Due to the worldwide proliferation of this sweetener, you would be hard pressed not to have any in your diet. Still, you should try to limit the amount that you consume. Just reading the ingredients of the food you consume will help you remove most of the HFCS from your diet. Pursuing this goal will also limit the amount of processed foods that you consume, which will give you additional health benefits.

Complex Carbohydrates

For most people, your diet should consist primarily of complex carbohydrates. This allows your body a slow, steady stream of usable calories. This helps to regulate your energy levels as well as your mood. There has been a tendency in a lot of popular diets lately to overemphasize the consumption of protein. This is not necessary for your body's needs and can be harmful to your body in the long run. Your body breaks down excess protein into carbohydrates and gets rid of the urea through your kidneys and ultimately your urine. The broken down proteins are then repackaged into fats if enough of them exist. This gives people the false sense that they can consume as much protein as they want without getting fat, which is simply not the case. There is also the additional burden on the environment to produce many protein-rich foods.

The amount of complex carbohydrates necessary for one's diet depends on their lifestyle as well as their genetics, but around 50% is a good guideline. It is up to you to determine what percentage works for you. I would suggest you experiment with different levels but also listen to your body. We tend to desire the types of foods that we need. So if you are craving carbs, you probably need to increase (slowly) the amount you consume. Some sources of these carbs are listed below.

Sources of Complex Carbohydrates

- Beans (i.e., pinto, navy, lima, garbanzo)
- Brown or wild rice
- Lentils
- Oatmeal
- Peas
- Potatoes
- Quinoa
- Whole-grain bread

The list above is just a sample of the available complex carbohydrates, but it should give you a good idea of what to look for. Many foods contain a mixture of complex and simple carbohydrates, such as bananas, apples, or grapefruit. These foods can provide a quick energy boost in addition to the longer energy release. You will need to develop a diet that will provide for your needs, but it should always have a core of complex carbohydrates.

Fat

Fat gets a bad rap from the media, but it is an essential part of your diet, especially for developing bodies. Fat provides cushioning between the various components of your body, is necessary for brain health, and can be converted into carbohydrates for long-term energy. But as with all good things, you want to consume fat in moderation. Some fats are better to consume than others, and you should remember that when deciding which types to consume, simply look at the number of grams of fat. The different types of fats are gone over in detail in the following sections so you can determine which kinds you want to consume or avoid.

Trans Fats

Trans fats (a specific type of unsaturated fat) are regarded as the "bad" fats. There are a lot of different studies out there, but the consensus is that trans fats are bad for your health. They are generally not found in nature, which is a good clue that they are probably not good to put in your body. There are small amounts of trans fats in animals such as cows, and these fats are considered just as bad as those produced chemically. But the amounts of trans fats that occur naturally are generally low and do not present the same concerns as those industrially produced. One of the benefits of trans fats is that they generally store longer than other kinds of fats. This long-term storage ability and desirable melting properties are why they are used by the industry.

Trans fats are considered harmful because they tend to increase bad cholesterol (low density lipids or LDL) and lower the good cholesterol (high density lipids or HDL). This leads to the accumulation of plaque in your arteries and can eventually lead to a heart attack or stroke. Although there are some people who can consume trans fats on a regular basis and show no heart disease, the overall danger factor is leading to fewer and fewer of these showing up in products on our shelves. There is even a strong push to outlaw the industrialized production of these fats. A wide variety of other health issues have been linked to trans fats too, although they have not been studied in nearly as much depth as heart disease. In any case, you should watch out for trans fats and try to keep them out of your diet as much as possible.

Saturated Fats

These are fats that could potentially be harmful to your body in that they have a direct impact on increasing the LDL cholesterol in your body according to many studies. However, it seems that this may be worse in some saturated fats than in others. Unlike trans fats, saturated fats occur quite commonly in nature and can take up a significant part of your caloric intake if you are not careful.

Common Sources of Saturated Fats

- Bacon
- Butter
- Cocoa butter (found in chocolate)
- Coconut milk
- Coconut oil
- Cottonseed oil
- Palm kernel oil
- Red meat
- Sausage
- Whole milk

Unsaturated Fats

These are the fats that are considered good for you. Some of them can even help improve your cholesterol levels and are considered good for your heart. For example, olive oil increases your HDL levels, which helps to decrease your LDL levels. Omega-3 fatty acids (from fish) helps to lower triglycerides. While unsaturated fats may be good for you, it is still not a good idea to overdo them, plus they are still as high in calories as other fats.

Common Sources of Unsaturated Fats

- Avocado oil
- Canola oil
- Fish (anchovies, mackerel, salmon, sardines, tuna)
- Nuts
- Olives
- Safflower oil
- Seeds
- Soybean oil

Proteins

Proteins are the primary building blocks for your body. The proteins your body uses are made of twenty-one amino acids that are divided into two groups, commonly called essential and nonessential. The nonessential ones are still required by the body to function effectively, but they can be synthesized internally from other amino acids (although some amino acids require certain other proteins to begin with). This means that you can take other amino acids that already exist within your body and change them into the nonessential ones.

Essential amino acids must be acquired via your diet. This is especially problematic for vegetarians and vegans because their diet usually does not contain all the essential amino acids. A few grains contain all of the essential amino acids (such as the now quite popular quinoa). but it takes a special effort to make sure that these amino acids are consumed in adequate quantities so the body has all of the amino acids that it needs.

There is a trend to try diets that include far more protein than your body needs. These diets do seem to have short-term weight loss results, but for the most part the participants in these diets tend to gain back all the weight that they lost and even more. There are probably many reasons for this, but I believe the body mainly starts craving the carbs that it is missing, and when it finally does get them it does the best it can to store them up as fat.

In any case, consuming more protein than you need just turns the excess into carbohydrates and potentially into fat. Your body has no method of storing extra protein as protein, so it is a use-it-or-lose-it situation. The process creates a lot of urea (the stuff that turns urine yellow), which can have negative effects on the body. If you do decide to participate in one of these protein-focused diets, make sure that you consume adequate amounts of water and do not take additional protein supplements. Unless you are involved in an extremely rigorous workout routine that breaks down your muscles, your protein needs are quite minimal. Just think of them as building blocks. If you are not building anything, they just end up getting flushed down the toilet.

Vitamins And Minerals

There are a ton of vitamin and mineral supplements available that make all sorts of claims about how much better they will make your life. I have found that you only need to consume enough vitamins and minerals to meet your body's needs. The rest are just surplus that create a burden on your kidneys or liver and get sent out of your body. I am not pro vitamin supplements, but I am not totally against them either. I think you should try to get your vitamins through your food when possible and to supplement when you cannot.

You can increase the amount of nutrients you get by not overcooking your food and by choosing foods that are high in a variety of nutrients. This generally means eating a wide variety of foods, since no one food contains everything your body needs. Most foods are high in one or two nutrients but generally lack other nutrients or have them in very low amounts.

Most of us think taking vitamins and minerals or consuming them through certain foods is a good thing, and in most cases that is true. However, you can overdo taking vitamins, and in rare cases this can even cause death. This situation is exacerbated if you are on a strict diet or fasting as well as not drinking enough water. Water-soluble vitamins are generally safer than fat-soluble ones since they are processed more quickly. But even if you do not take enough to kill yourself, overdosing vitamins can cause a host of other issues, such as kidney stones, hot flashes, excessive bleeding (hemorrhaging), birth defects, nerve problems, and interference with medications you may be taking.

Water-Soluble Vitamins

Water-soluble vitamins pass through the body rather rapidly. In fact, if you drink too much water you could run low on them. This means that you need to take water-soluble vitamins on a regular basis (preferably through food but through supplements if you cannot obtain adequate quantities via your diet). On the plus side, if you take too many of these vitamins they are quickly eliminated from your body through urine. This may affect the color and/or smell of your urine. While this is not an indication of bad health, it does mean that your kidneys are working much harder than they need to. The benefits/dangers of overworking your kidneys are still up for debate, but if you are having any sort of kidney issues you should be cautious of taking too many water-soluble vitamins.

List of Water-Soluble Vitamins

- Vitamin B1 (Thiamine)
- Vitamin B2 (Riboflavin)
- Vitamin B3 (Niacin)

- Vitamin B5 (Pantothenic Acid)
- Vitamin B6 (Pyridoxine)
- Vitamin B9 (Folic Acid)
- Vitamin B12 (Cobalamin)
- Vitamin C

Fat-Soluble Vitamins

Vitamins that can be stored in fat do not have to be consumed as frequently as their water-soluble counterparts. This means it easier to get them through your diet, and supplements are not nearly as important. Trying to get all of your vitamins via your diet will ensure that you are eating the proper amount of fruits and vegetables as well as a diverse diet. The fact that you do not have to consume fat-soluble vitamins as often as water-soluble ones is both good and bad. Excessive amounts of vitamins consumed end up staying in your system much longer. With the water-soluble ones you can just drink a lot of water to get rid of the excess, but with fat-soluble ones you have to actually use them to get rid of them, and that might take a while depending on how much you are consuming. Most people do not have to worry about this, but if you are taking excessive amounts of these vitamins via supplements, you might want to check the levels of the vitamins listed below.

List of Fat-Soluble Vitamins

- Vitamin A
- Vitamin D
- Vitamin E
- Vitamin K

Basics Of A Good Diet

The essentials of a good diet vary from person to person. Your genetics play a major role in the types of foods you should consume. Your daily activity also determines the kinds of calories you should be consuming. Even though each person differs in their dietary requirements, there are some basics that apply to your diet regardless of your genetics. These general guidelines are shown below.

Eating Checklist

- Eat a variety of foods.
- Eat several smaller meals a day rather than a few large meals.
- Eat when you wake up or shortly thereafter since your body has been fasting during rest.
- Avoid eating large amounts of food before bed, especially those high in calories.
- Avoid overly processed foods and try to consume raw foods when possible.
- Fiber is an absolute must for the proper functioning of your digestive system.
- Avoid excess amounts of alcohol, especially binge drinking.
- Avoid drugs that can cause damage to your body. This includes most drugs if taken for an extended period of time.
- Avoid drugs and foods that are addictive.

CHAPTER 3: SPIRITUAL SPOKE BASICS

The spiritual spoke is the hardest spoke to measure but may be the most important one. If your spiritual spoke is damaged, it is very hard to keep the rest of your wheel from falling apart. Visual inspection and/or physical measurements can easily determine if someone is out of shape and their physical spoke is damaged, but it is often hard to determine the health of their spiritual spoke visually. From the outside they can appear happy and content, but inside they are falling apart. Without having a deep, personal connection with that person, it may be impossible to determine their spiritual wellness.

There is no one path to spiritual strength. For some people this strength can be found by participating in one of the organized religions of the world. This book is far too limited to address each of these groups in detail. Religion can be a valuable tool for strengthening your spiritual spoke but is not for everyone. Luckily, it is not the only way to strengthen your spiritual essence. With or without religion, you must maintain your spiritual spoke to make your wheel whole and able to withstand the rigors of rolling through the world.

Worship

Religion has been with us since the beginning of history and probably much longer. There are many religions in the world, each with their own merits. Your beliefs are your personal choice and adherence to them can benefit your spiritual well-being. Worship can bring a community together and help strengthen you throughout your journey in this world. The people who worship with you can provide spiritual support that can bolster your goals to become a better you.

Whatever your beliefs, there is a religion that is appropriate to your needs. Even atheists have churches these days. They have acknowledged that everyone needs a place to call home and that community is important for a well-rounded individual. I hope that you will consider this in your journey and decide whether religion is appropriate for you.

Spiritual Spoke Constructors

Your spirit needs uplifting and strengthening to help you handle life's inevitable stresses. Nobody is immune to the ups and downs of life. If your spirit is strong, you are more prepared to handle these stressors and keep them from damaging your wheel. This section will cover some of the actions that can reinforce your spiritual spoke, making you happier and more content during even the most difficult times.

Acceptance

Most of us spend a lot of time and energy on things we cannot change. We stress over them, complain about them, and dream that they will change by themselves. But there are some things we just cannot change no matter how hard we or anyone else tries. Acceptance of this fact will help you make peace with what you cannot change and will make you happier and healthier. It will also free your mind from contemplating your future, full of endless possibilities, and trying to perform impossible tasks so it can better handle your day-to-day responsibilities. Acceptance will also give you more time in your day to spend with those you care about and to focus on activities that benefit you.

To find peace with the past is the first acceptance goal. There is absolutely nothing you can do to change what has already happened. You can remember it and learn from it, but you gain nothing by trying to change it. You will know you are wasting your valuable resources if you hear yourself saying phrases that begin "if only," "I wish that," or "I should have." If you catch yourself using these words, stop and think about whether speaking this way benefits you at all. If not (and almost certainly it does not), why spend your time and energy speaking like this? It can only hinder you from appreciating the present and achieving the goals you set.

The second acceptance goal is to realize and accept who you are. This means coming to terms with the capabilities and limitations you were born with. Everyone has a set of positive attributes they can use throughout their lives. You will be naturally better at some parts of life than at other parts. Nobody is good at everything, but you can definitely work on improving most of your talents.

It is natural to feel envious over talents or skills you lack and wish you were more capable. For example, you may never be able to dunk a basketball, be a chess champion, or run a marathon no matter what you do. But whether you can or cannot does not make you a better or worse person. These are simply things you can or cannot do. They are just activities, and you give them the weight you want to give them.

Sometimes others like family members or friends might push us, but you can choose how you react to this pressure. Wishing you could do something you will never be able to or working toward something you really do not want is a waste of time and energy. You are capable of so many wonderful things no matter who you are that if you just focus on what you can do instead of what you cannot do, there is no limit to what you can accomplish.

Whether the obstacle is physical or mental, accept who you are and try to focus on being the best person you can be without comparing yourself to others. The only one you should compete with is yourself, at least in the game of life. Holding this attitude takes some training, but once you master it you can unlock true happiness.

Gratitude

As we progress through life, we often focus on the negatives, or more specifically the parts of our lives that need to be fixed or altered. This is pretty much true with the rest of life as well. The news rarely focuses on what is actually working but gravitates towards the negative. The problems get the most attention, and we end up ignoring the parts of our life that are going well.

For example, if a community has gone years without a major crime, you will never hear about it on the news unless a murder or other heinous crime occurs there. Then you will hear about how a "peaceful" community was destroyed by such an act. The truth is that most of us are surrounded by things we should be grateful for. Most of us have been spoiled and fail to appreciate even the basic necessities of life, taking them for granted. We should be grateful for some things each day, such as

- Having enough food to eat
- Having clean water
- Having air to breathe
- Being alive
- Having shelter to keep us from harm

If the basic needs are met, the rest of life is just extra even though we usually find it hard to appreciate this fact. The media focuses on very small fragments of our society and makes us think these fragments represent the whole. This behavior gets the media ratings and makes them money. Our very nature is to be rubberneckers. In essence, we are built to focus on what is not normal in our environment. This trait helped us avoid dangers in the past but can also prevent us from appreciating the enjoyable parts of life.

A healthy portion of your day should consist of appreciating all the good things in your life instead of focusing on the negatives that want to consume your time and energy. This appreciation will keep your spiritual spoke strong and improve your lifelong happiness. By focusing on the positives in your life, you can gain a more balanced outlook and support yourself through any difficult times.

Sometimes you will not have good health, but when you do, you will appreciate it even more and do what you can to keep it. Being more positive in general is good for your overall health and keeps many of the world's negative effects at bay. You can channel the energy you gather from being positive into making more changes that help you reach your goals. This is not always easy to do, and you will slip up at times. But if you wake up every day and realize you are grateful for what you have, you will be well on your way to achieving your goals in life.

Exercise: Gratitude

Every morning when you wake up, think of at least three things you are grateful for. This can be as simple as having a comfortable bed to sleep in, having food to look forward to for breakfast, or if you are lucky, waking up in a household where there are people who care about you. If you just look around a bit, you will easily find things you are grateful for, especially if you can put your troubles aside for a while and focus only on the positives.

Do this exercise for a few weeks at first, then turn it into a regular practice. Personally, I find it easier to think of everything I am grateful for at night before I go to bed, mainly because after the alarm clock goes off in the morning it is a race to get to work. So although morning would be best, use any time of day that works for you. Just make sure to take time to be thankful for all the good things this wonderful world has to offer even during the difficult times we all endure.

Taking Breaks

It is very true that you need to take breaks from your everyday life. This mean breaks from work, kids, money stresses, and whatever else pulls on you. Of course, saying that and doing it are two different things. Life gets very full if you let it with things that are not truly important.

First, you should determine what is truly important and what can wait or what can be eliminated. Unimportant tasks have a way of taking over life and filling it up. You have to find a way to eliminate these tasks. A simple example is to unsubscribe from email subscriptions that you don't value so you can reduce the clutter in your life. This doesn't take a lot of time to do but can save you hours and hours in the future.

Once you make the effort to take a break, try to truly unwind and forget about your troubles. This is something I find really hard to do. I try to relax, and the troubles of the world come flooding in. I feel guilty for relaxing even though I know I need to so I can be a better person for those around me. I let work creep into my head and focus on issues that could easily wait until I return. I worry about how my kids and family are doing. I worry about bills that need to be paid and on and on. Clearing the mind takes practice and willpower. You will get better at it. Know that it is good for you and that in the end it will be good for the people you care about.

Breaks do not have to come in multi-day excursions, although those are essential to your mental and spiritual well-being. Breaks can come in short bursts through the day just as well. I try to take small breaks often when I am working. Taking short walks helps me with this. I can just concentrate on the walk itself and my surroundings, freeing my mind from tasks I have to take care of at work and challenges outside of work.

Many people find meditation helpful, though I have found it

difficult. As soon as I try to meditate, my mind wanders within a minute. The silence deafens me and my heartbeat starts to sound loud. My mind goes to anything it can rather than allowing me to just clear it and rest. Many of you will relate to this situation. To me nothing is harder than doing nothing, but sometimes that is exactly what is most needed.

Connecting With Your Community

There are a multitude of ways to connect with your community. Humans are social animals and need connections with other human beings to make our lives complete. Some of this can be through family, but we also need to reach out and connect with those around us: the people we work with, the people who live next to us, and the people we see on a regular basis.

This involves more effort than you might think because you are not going to see eye to eye with everyone you interact with. This is to be expected and can help you grow to be a more complete person. Life is challenging, and getting along with people you disagree with is one of the biggest challenges. On the positive side, you will also find friends you can rely upon during difficult times. Even some of the people you find it difficult to deal with will come around when times are tough.

It is amazing how many people do not know the people who live next to them these days. We have become isolated in our houses, walling off everything around us. We might be on a first-name basis with people halfway around the world, but we cannot name the people who live next door.

Connecting With Nature

With the urbanization of societies across the globe it has gotten much more difficult for many of us to enjoy nature. Just a short 100 or even 50 years ago, most people lived in rural areas and in small communities where most people knew each other. Living in urban areas is a new and not altogether healthy phenomenon dictated by many factors such as the population explosion and a desire for the material benefits a city can provide. There are other benefits too, such as access to better education and hospitals, but as with most benefits, there is a cost. Those eons of living outdoors have permeated our DNA and our spirits, and when we leave the outdoors we leave a part of us behind. As human beings, we need a connection with the natural world around us to be truly whole.

The kind of city you live in and where you live within that city determines how the lack of being in nature affects you. Some cities have had the forethought to plan natural areas scattered throughout the residential zones. In certain cases they did this regardless of how much money they could get from developers. The founders and planners of those cities realized how important it was for us to have these natural areas to enjoy, and more importantly for the people who will come after us as well. Being around nature somehow brings us a sense of calm and happiness. It is something that cannot be truly expressed with words and must be experienced in person, but we all need it at the very core of our being. It makes us realize that we are just small parts of an intricately connected universe. Stepping out into nature is the only way to truly see life in action and know that you are just one tiny component in the web of life.

If you are stuck in a world where nature is absent or in short supply, you can try to bring the outdoors in. There are a host of different ways to do this even if you cannot spend a lot of time taking care of the life that you bring indoors. Inviting plants and animals (if you can) into your life provides you with a host of benefits for your spirit, mind, and body. The simple act of petting a cat or a dog has been shown to lower your blood pressure. Animals can give you a sense of belonging and bring true happiness. Plants generate fresh oxygen and lower the carbon dioxide in the nearby area, helping you breathe easier and think more clearly. Plants and animals should not and do not replace human interaction, but they do add a different and helpful component to your life.

Being in a truly sterile environment will leave an empty spot in your spiritual spoke that will eventually cause your wheel to suffer. Even a few small succulents in your office or your apartment can make a big difference, and they need very little care. I have found that taking care of fish helps relieve my stress even though it requires a bit of attention. Of course, once you start with a few small plants and fish, you may find yourself getting more and more to take care of. The life you bring into your sphere of being will rely on you and you will begin to rely on it. It will be work and there will be failures, but there will also be growth and caring as you develop bonds with the beings that exist in your life. These bonds strengthen you and they strengthen the lives that you are taking care of.

One of the most important things you can do for your health and your sanity is to unplug every once in a while. Electronics have taken over our lives and it is not a healthy transition. When we are not in front of a computer we are on our phones or sitting in front of our televisions. There are literally hundreds of television channels and an unlimited number of web sites to consume our time and our spirits. If you are like me, it is very hard to get away from these electronic devices. It is how I make my living, it is how I stay in touch with the people I care about, and it is how I entertain myself when I get some rare downtime.

We have become trapped by the electronic revolution, but we are not digital creatures and we were not meant to be strapped to these electronic devices. They were meant to aid us, not enslave us, but that is how they have evolved. We are slaves to these things. In order to prevent a total takeover, you must put these instruments aside and venture out into the wilderness on occasion and cut the electronic cord. This might seem harsh at first, but it is necessary for you to prevent a total takeover. We all need a break from the constant pressure of being on all the time. The never-ending email, the constant social newsfeeds, and the relentless pressure of sales and marketing trying to get your attention all exert mental pressure.

Get out and enjoy life. You can go sailing to a remote location that lacks internet or cell service. You can travel to an exotic location and unwind on a quiet beach with nothing to do but turn over every once in a while. You can take a hike into the wilderness and turn your cell phone off, knowing that whatever it is, it can wait until you return. Email, texts and whatever else can wait on you. You must take care of yourself before you can take care of others, and sometimes that means cutting the cord.

Make Room For Happiness

Remember when you were a little kid and something small would make you so happy. It could have been a balloon, a cloud, or even a funny noise. Being happy is good for you. As we get older, those expressions of happiness are suppressed. As our worries mount and the past traumas build, it becomes harder and harder to be truly happy. You might even feel guilty for being happy. When you laugh you might look around as if something is going to come down and destroy your moment of happiness. This is normal behavior but it is not healthy behavior. You have to allow yourself to be happy. Make room for laughter and smiling and being silly. Life is so short. It is a blink in the eye of the universe and you need to be happy when you can.

Being happy is more a state of mind than anything else. If you focus on being miserable then you will always be miserable. Some days really, really suck and there is no way around it. That is just part of life. However, most days are a mixture of moments that allow for you to be happy if you only take time to notice them. Many times in my life I have been down and found happiness in the simple things during my day. For example, a beautiful sunset on my way home from a long commute has made me happy and allowed me to put a smile on my face. There are many other avenues to find happiness. It can be something as simple as the smell of a flower, the taste of a delicious meal or the greeting of someone you care about. You need to search out these moments of happiness and incorporate them into your daily routine.

The biggest hurdle to your happiness is probably you. Most of us find it difficult to allow ourselves to be happy for one reason or another. You will have to find a way to overcome this hurdle if you want your wheel to be whole. You deserve happiness in your life no matter who you are or what you have done in your past. You will have to let that go temporarily so you can allow some room in your life for being happy. If you can do this, your path to a longer and more fulfilling life will be much easier.

Unplug

It seems like everybody is connected all the time now. This is definitely not a healthy way to live. This is just not my opinion but has been proven in multiple studies showing that people who spend more time connected feel worse about themselves. The world is a huge place and there are billions of people in it. It is impossible to keep up with everything and there really is no benefit in trying. You should keep up with how the world is doing to a certain extent, but you should be more concerned about how you are doing than how others are doing.

I recommend taking dedicated time to unplug from all electronic communication methods to get the full benefit from being unplugged. Humankind has survived for millennia without being plugged in, so I think you can survive a few days without this artificial artifact that is attempting to take over our lives. Time and time again I see people taking selfies or posting that they are someplace that they perceive to be cool or important. For the most part, social media posters do not even take the time to enjoy the places they are posting about. They simply want to brag about how they were there so they can try to make themselves feel better.

My question to these people is, how can you enjoy a sunset if you are trying to take a picture of yourself pretending you are enjoying it? I do not blame these individuals. They are simply a reflection of how our society has changed to one that thrives on instant gratification rather than lasting accomplishments that take time, energy and focus.

Our lives are composed of fleeting moments that you have to

be present in to truly appreciate and enjoy. There is time to reflect upon them once they happen. Most of life is about showing up, and when you do, you need to make sure you have shown up in the truest sense. We are bombarded with a constant influx of stimuli that our brains were not designed to handle. It is built into our DNA because it is essential that we react quickly to certain outside stimuli so we can decide whether we should flee or fight as a danger presents itself.

Unfortunately, this quick reaction to new information has been turned against us and used for marketing and manipulation. Corporations and politicians use this technique to attempt to control us. Whenever there is a situation we need to focus on to solve, they use these distracting techniques so that we end up focusing on the minutiae instead of what should really matter in our world. This is similar to how magicians use distraction to perform their various tricks, but much more insidious.

You will make your spiritual spoke much stronger if you do take breaks from being bombarded by distracting and useless information all day long in the myriad of available ways. Cutting the cord makes it easier to be your own person and to make your own decisions. Following everyone else's rules means you will end up just like them. The whole goal of this book is to help you break free from these chains and be your own person. So, be different and start judging yourself and not everyone else in the world, for that is a battle you can never win.

Spiritual Spoke Destroyers

There are many things in life we have to deal with that will attempt to bring us down. I call these spiritual spoke destroyers. Although life requires you to deal with these elements, you do not have to succumb to their pressures. Life is not fair. Losers win the lottery and hardworking people get the shaft. That is how it is, but you do not have to let this fact ruin your life. You can make your life better by removing the spoke destroyers, these highly negative elements. You cannot control what happens to you, but you can control how you react. Life is too short to spend your time on petty things, so try to make the most of the time you have. Use this book to help you identify and work to remove whatever is detrimental in your life.

Hate

Allowing hate to control your life is one of the quickest ways to destroy your spirit and one of the most harmful to you. It is also one of the hardest emotions to control once it gets a grip on you. Almost all of us allow ourselves to fall into the trap of hate – it is one of our most basic instincts. Allowing hate to gain roots and grow within us will only harm us and empower others to gain control over us. Remember, those who can control your reactions can control how you feel.

The object of hate could be a person, a group, or a situation, but the outcome is the same: You are allowing external influences to control how you feel and react. Hate can make you act and think in ways you normally would consider irrational or even insane if you observed them in someone else. In severe cases hate and hate-fueled reactions can cause incalculable, permanent damage to you and to those around you. Sadly, the people we harm in these cases are usually the ones we care the most about.

One sure sign that hate is controlling your life is that the object of your hate will come to the forefront of your mind and start to appear in your dreams. An occasional dream is generally not a concern, but if it is a recurring theme, you need to take measures to identify and control this hate before it turns into a full-blown obsession.

Beware the hate mongers! Hatred in any form is detrimental to your well-being despite the righteous behavior that you might be tempted to champion. The most dangerous hate mongers are the ones who believe they stand behind a "noble" cause, which people tend to cling to so they can feel better about their own behaviors or assuage some real or imaginary guilt. These noble causes tend to be a religion, an oppressed group, or racism but can take the form of almost any cause which has a "righteous" component. While purporting to support this cause, its supporters foment an attitude of hate and division, often undermining the very cause they support.

Hate takes many different forms, and various groups exist that are openly hate groups. These more overt groups are easy to identify, and if you happen to be a part of one of these groups, you are destroying your spirit. Whatever organization or cause you might be behind, take a long, hard look at the energy you are putting into it. If that energy is positive and uplifting, then you are helping others and yourself. But if it is negative, you need to make sure you are doing the right things for the right reasons. Do not let yourself be drawn into the witch-hunt mentality that is still pervasive in our society.

You should try to understand the causes of any hateful feelings you are having, then try to control them once you have identified them. This works best if you start off being a well-balanced whole person, but this very hate may be unbalancing you. To beat hate you must remove the emotional connection and try to analyze it objectively. Simply reminding yourself that you are allowing the object of hate to control you will often help. You will have to rise above these feelings of hate.

Choosing to let hate go does not mean you have to agree with or approve of what you hate. It means that you are not letting the object of hate inspire irrational actions. If you hate someone, try being nice and pleasant to them, since they are probably the ones who need it the most. When you find yourself dwelling on the object of hate, try doing something you enjoy or spending time with someone you love. Talk to someone about how you feel and how it is affecting you.

The cure for hate is love. Even though that might sound overly simple, it is very hard for most of us to embody. Just keep trying. Eventually you will be able to overcome these feelings, or at least get them under control so you can proceed with your own life.

Idol Worship

Idol worship is irrational admiration of an object or person. It could be a mystical godlike being or a mundane human being who has been thrust upon some imaginary pedestal either in society or just in your own mind. The worst thing about idol worship is that most people don't even realize that they are doing it, much less the damage it can cause. Even if you do not recognize your idol worship, others around you probably will.

If you are lucky enough to have a true friend, they will try to point it out and help you realize it is an issue. If you are a well-balanced person, you are much less likely to have this problem in the first place. It is directly related to a perceived deficiency in your own self-worth. We see attributes in the object of our worship that we think are desirable and wish we had, then we transfer those desires into irrational wants that progress to idolization of that person or object. We then begin to assign that object attributes they truly do not have. People are all just flawed, imperfect human beings, nothing more. That is perfectly fine, and expecting anything else is one of the quickest ways to disappointment.

It is fine to admire a person for skills or talents they have. If you want to benefit from this admiration, you can use it to inspire you to better yourself. Remember that life should not be a spectator sport and it is up to you to decide if you are going to be a player. The most common idols of today are those in sports, music, and movies. We are so inundated by the media that we fall into traps of believing these people have greater than human attributes when they are simply fault-filled individuals like the rest of us.

Each person needs to look deep inside themselves to find their own self-worth, for each and every one of us is capable of greatness in our own way. True self-worth cannot be gained by the words or admiration of others. It can only be gained from within. If you are not at peace with yourself, you can never truly gain that peace from the thoughts and actions of others. Just remember that every one of us is worthy and important.

Mild cases of idol worship may simply consist of following someone's career very closely, buying a lot of products associated with that person, and talking about the person daily. Severe cases could involve going into debt, ignoring your mate and friends, and trying to imitate that person. In any case, idol worship is unhealthy for the spirit and therefore detrimental to the wheel which is you.

None of us are perfect. We are all just humans trying to make it through this journey of life. Don't assume someone is better than you and that his or her life is better. The most beneficial thing you can do is to focus on making your own life better. There are billions of people on the planet, so comparing yourself to others is a futile task. Make decisions you will be proud of in the future and do the best you can. No one can ask more.

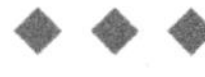

Jealousy

Jealousy at its roots is simply wanting what someone else has instead of them having it. You should always be happy for someone else for doing well as long as they are not prospering at your expense. This is a very hard task and it must come from deep within, since you are fighting a very basic instinct that exists not only in humans but also in primates and possibly other animals too. Jealousy exists within you because you are not content with your own situation in life. Typically, you might be content until you see that someone else has it better than you do. Only you have the power to change whether you are jealous or not. Learning not to be jealous takes considerable effort and is something you may have to revisit regularly. It will take time and effort but is within everyone's grasp.

Next time you see someone excel at something, go up and

congratulate them and try be honest about it. This will be especially hard in situations where you feel you might have been slighted, such as with a job promotion or an award given. Despite the effort it might take, try to be happy for them. Being jealous only consumes energy and time that you could be using to better yourself so you can achieve the accolades and rewards you think you deserve. If you cannot avoid having these feelings of jealousy, try to use that energy in a positive manner so you can do better in the future. If you let jealousy turn inward, it will eat at your spirit and eventually your mind and body too.

The ultimate goal is to look only at your own life and therefore compete only against yourself. If you study hard and do well on a test, be happy about it. Don't worry about the person next to you. If your neighbors get a brand-new car and you still drive a ten- or twenty-year-old clunker, be happy for them. It may be hard at first, but the more complete a person you become, the easier it will be.

Deceit

It is important to try to be honest as much as you can. When you start down the road of deceit, it is hard to get off it. One lie will lead to another, and eventually you will lose track of where one starts and the other ends. In practice, telling the truth all the time can be difficult. There are many reasons you might be propelled to lie, sometimes from good intentions. You may refrain from telling the truth to save yourself or someone else from harm. Often we are punished for telling the truth, especially in close relationships. The way to solve this problem is to refrain from doing anything you would have a problem telling the truth about. This does not mean you will never do anything you feel ashamed or embarrassed about, but that you try to live a life you can be proud of.

The most important person to be honest with is yourself. If you can't be truthful with yourself, it is impossible to be honest with anyone else. The second most important person is your life mate. You must try to be honest with your life mate. It will be hard at times because you may not want to hurt them or you don't want them to be angry with you. In turn you must let your partner be honest with you and understand that they are human and also make mistakes. If you do your best to be good to yourself and your partner, your life will be rich indeed.

Narcissism

We all want to feel good about ourselves and to think we are important. It is important to love yourself, but self-admiration can be carried too far. Everyone is important and valuable, but no one is perfect. No matter how smart you are, there is someone smarter. No matter how good-looking you think you are, you are ugly to someone. There is always someone better. Even if you happen to be the absolute best at something, it is ephemeral.

Narcissism not only hurts you, but it can also be detrimental to those around you. By constantly harping on your attributes you can make others feel bad about not meeting this artificially introduced standard. Let others praise you, and be happy in knowing you are doing your best.

Self-Loathing

This is the opposite of narcissism and is far more common. Self-loathing can completely destroy a person's mind, body, and spirit. You must consider yourself important and valuable. Everyone deserves a chance in this world, and you have to allow yourself that chance. If you put yourself down, how can you expect anyone else to respect you?

Often we allow events to make us hate ourselves. Never let someone else's actions make you feel bad about yourself. If you didn't do the act or cause it to happen, don't blame yourself. Blame never solved anything anyhow. It is just used by others to make themselves feel better. If someone of the same race, sex, or religion as you does a heinous act, it doesn't make you any worse or better, and you are in no way responsible. This doesn't mean you should condone such an act. You should be the first person to condemn it, but don't take the blame on yourself.

Physical appearance can often lead to self-loathing. You shouldn't think less of yourself just because you don't fit a certain physical mold or type. We allow ourselves to let the media and peer pressure determine what is beautiful and what is ugly. Beauty should come from the inside. If your friends make you feel bad about how you look, maybe they aren't really your friends. You can improve the situation by taking care of yourself and feeling good about your body, and this will strongly influence how others perceive you. Ultimately, if you are happy you won't care what others think about you.

Blame

No one wants to blame themselves for their problems. It is always someone else's fault. Blame is a crutch that needs to be thrown away. Even if it is someone else's fault, spending time and effort blaming someone doesn't help you. Your current situation is what it is. You can blame society, your job, or the people around you, but you still have to be responsible for your actions. If you are not happy with your life you have to change it. If you don't change it, you are letting others control how you spend your life and you have no one to blame but yourself.

Intimidation

Intimidation is using some means of control over a person to make them do something. It may be money or physical strength or blackmail. It can manifest itself as physical or mental abuse, or even sexual abuse. Whatever the manifestation of intimidation, it is detrimental to your spirit if you use it and will eventually catch up to you. When you intimidate you make an enemy, giving rise to fear and resentment. People do not like to be coerced into anything, even if it is something they would normally do under other circumstances. People want to be respected and thanked for their efforts. If a person does not want to do something, you need to respect that.

People often resort to intimidation because they are not whole people. One of the three spokes is lacking, and through intimidation they try to make up for that lack. They may feel that they are weak in body and use money or position to try and make others feel lesser. They may also feel less intelligent than those around them and try to use money and power to create the illusion of intelligence. These people also try to belittle intelligent individuals by focusing on any negative trait or difference they can find. The biggest reason someone uses intimidation is that they have been intimidated in the past, probably at an early age. This damages the spirit and creates a circle of intimidation that is hard to break. When someone tries to intimidate you, try to understand where that person is coming from. Don't let them bully you if you can avoid it, but also don't let them turn you into a bully. That is the real way to defeat them and to help yourself as well.

Excessive Worrying

With news now covering the entire world, there is always something to worry about, whether locally or far away. You can worry about almost anything. You can worry about world hunger, or you can worry about whether it will rain. The only thing this accomplishes is strain on the heart and spirit. This doesn't mean you shouldn't be concerned about the problems in life, but don't dwell on them. If you are truly concerned you can find a way to help. If for some reason you can't help, you shouldn't worry at all. You might as well worry about when the sun burns out 5 billion years from now.

Most excessive worry consists of worrying about others. If you are going to expend energy worrying, you should worry about yourself first and foremost. Then you can channel some of that energy into positive results. You must first realize you are worrying, then decide to make a change. You could decide to do more work, more exercise, less eating, or anything else that will help you attain the goals you have set in life.

Don't let worry keep you from being happy. Everyone needs happiness in life. It feeds and nurtures the spirit, while excessive worry denies the spirit the very sustenance it needs to survive.

Overindulging

At first thought, you might wonder how overindulging could destroy your spirit, though it is fairly easy to see how it can affect your physical and mental spokes. On further inspection it becomes obvious that these excesses can destroy the very core of your spirit. If all you focus on is catering to your carnal desires, the whole person will disintegrate. Maintaining the person as a whole takes work and determination. It's true that being a whole person includes allowing yourself to be happy, but don't become hedonistic. Do not drink until you are drunk, do not eat until you are gorged, and do not care only about your own needs. That is a short-sighted view of how to obtain happiness and can only lead to a situation in which nothing you do will bring you the feelings of fulfillment you crave. Only by nurturing and maintaining your spirit can you achieve the desired result.

Hedonists are only concerned about their own well-being and do not care about the consequences of their actions to others, or even the long-term damage to themselves. While you might feel good pursuing hedonism in the moment, the damage incurred can be cumulative. You can lose friends, estrange your family and incur ill will from your neighbors. Eventually you become an empty shell and cannot feel happy no matter what you digest, smoke, drink, or have sex with. True happiness comes from within and cannot be gained from hedonistic acts. Those acts are simply illusions that disappear with the coming of the sun.

Contrary to what you might think after reading the last few paragraphs, I am in no way saying that you should not indulge at times in activities that bring you immediate gratification. There is nothing wrong with eating food that you find delicious, engaging in the pleasures of being intimate with another human being, or allowing yourself the delight of tasting your favorite vintage. Done in moderation, these activities can add to the enjoyment of life and reduce stress.

There are of course some activities (such as smoking cigarettes due to their addictive nature) that I would never recommend because the harmful effects outweigh any pleasure you would receive. So go out and enjoy the countless pleasures that life has to offer, but do so in a mindful way so as to avoid bringing harm to others or yourself, and your spirit will continue to support you.

Stress

Although stress can arise in and be felt in all three spokes, I decided to discuss it on the spiritual spoke, as I believe this is the most powerful place to address it. I like to think of stress as a bump in the road that can jar your wheel. Some of these bumps are small and a healthy wheel can handle them just fine, but some are deep potholes that damage the wheel and leave it in need of repair. Without those repairs your wheel becomes less capable of handling even the smaller bumps in life. Every little issue starts to seem insurmountable. Whatever the level of stress or the number of stressors you have, you must address how you handle stress if you want to achieve the goals of this book. Rich or poor, smart or uneducated, no matter what color or nationality, we all have to deal with stress in one way or another.

Stress should not be viewed as an evil to avoid at all costs. In fact, small amounts of stress are actually good for you. There is some truth to the adage of "what does not kill you makes you stronger," but this is only true if you don't permanently damage the spokes of your wheel. For example, losing a limb would cause stress you could live through but probably would not make you stronger. That is a graphic example, but it makes a point: You should not stress yourself past your limits on purpose. Dealing with the smaller stresses is great practice and develops skills that will protect your wheel from damage by the larger ones you will inevitably encounter.

The negative effects of stress are still being studied, but we know quite a bit about some of the side effects that long-term stress can cause:

Common Side Effects of Long-term Stress

- Memory loss
- Hardening of the arteries
- Weight gain due to insulin imbalance
- Weakened bones
- High blood pressure

These are just some of the known issues related to sustained cortisol levels. In a healthy scenario, you experience a stressful event (fender bender, unexpected bill, doctor's visit, etc.) and your cortisol levels spike. This is natural and expected and can even strengthen your spokes and ability to handle future stressors. The problem occurs when your stress levels stay elevated over long periods. Fortunately, most of the issues related to long-term stresses can be reversed – except for the memory loss, of course (though you may know more than you realize once you hone your mental skills). Your goal in maintaining your wheel is to identity these long-term stressors and do your best to minimize them, or at least let yourself take breaks from them.

Unfortunately, people often become accustomed to long-term stress. They fail to even see how the stress is affecting them until damage has been done (in some cases, very serious damage such as onset of Type 2 diabetes or Cushing's syndrome). Stressors such as not getting enough sleep; working or living in an environment that is too bright, smells bad, or is noisy; or living with someone argumentative all the time can cause chronically elevated cortisol levels. Sometimes it takes an outsider to see the stresses that are affecting you because you are so immersed in your own day-to-day activities.

Even small changes in your life can help alleviate the constant stress that so many of us have to deal with – changes as simple as changing the chair you sit in at work or even the one you relax in at home. If a chair does not support your body, it places stress on points along your spine and legs that may not be a big deal for a few days or weeks but eventually can cause joint pain, stooping, and nerve damage. Getting a proper chair is an easy solution that is often overlooked. Considering how much time most of us sit, we need to be in a position that does not cause any additional stress.

Another example is wearing ear plugs or noise-canceling earphones in a noisy environment so you can concentrate better. Certain types of noise produce stress, and that stress can be prolonged if this noise occurs regularly. Your conscious mind will try to ignore this noise eventually so it can function on other activities, but you are still being stressed. Your failure to consciously notice a stressor does not keep it from affecting you, and the damage at the end of the day is real.

Even though this is the spiritual section, so far we have mainly focused on physical and mental stresses. But these stresses, while not specifically spiritual in nature, do greatly affect your spirit nonetheless, and this is the component studies often overlook. These stresses can cause serious damage to your spiritual spoke, making you feel despondent and increasingly challenged to find the energy to remove these stressors. We gradually start to break down and accept these stresses as part of our lives and let them continue to destroy us.

Going beyond visible stressors, we also need to address spiritual stressors. We covered a lot of these under spiritual spoke destroyers, and they are a good place to start when looking for changes you can make to remove the factors keeping you from having the life you deserve. Sometimes this will require you to make dramatic changes that will affect those around you as well as yourself. You cannot keep doing the same things over and over again and expect different results. Life just doesn't work that way. Change is scary, and for a time after a major change it may feel uncomfortable, maybe even much worse than before the change. That is the nature of stress. We become comfortable far too easily with the negative aspects of our life, and when they are removed we feel loss and reluctance to let go, even if we and everyone around us know it is better in the long run.

Exercise: Examine Your Stressors

In this exercise you will examine the components in your life that cause your stress. The first step in solving a problem is to identify what the problem is, so ask yourself these questions.

1. Am I working too hard?
2. Am I getting enough sleep?
3. Am I allowing myself to take breaks to take care of myself?
4. Do I experience discomfort due to my environment (noise, physical discomfort, odors, lighting)?
5. Do I interact with people who lower my self-esteem on a regular basis?
6. Do I seek refuge in activities that hurt my body and mind, such as overeating or drinking too much?
7. Do I spend an inordinate amount of time performing activities I don't enjoy and don't find rewarding?

After you answer these questions, you will need to address anything you answered "yes" to and see if you can adjust your life to change each of those to a "no." Do this at least once a year, maybe around your birthday or at the beginning of the year. You should diligently address whatever problems you choose to work on. For example, I determined that my work environment was causing me stress due to noise and the length of the commute as well as a physically uncomfortable work environment (chair, desk, and lighting issues), so I worked out an arrangement that let me work from home part of the time. I had to hold firm to my position, but in the end I became a more productive employee and everybody won. I was happier to be at work and actually got more accomplished.

CHAPTER 4: MENTAL SPOKE BASICS

The human brain is one of the most complex structures we know about, with almost 100 billion interconnected neurons. This single organ weighing only a few pounds consumes around 25 percent of our daily calories. We are still trying to comprehend how it works even though we have made vast leaps in our knowledge of its substance and how its parts are connected. As we continue to understand more about the brain we can improve our ability to take care of it throughout our lives, enabling us to reach advanced years with fully functional mental capacity.

As one of the three spokes that makes you who you are, the mental spoke probably gets the least maintenance as we age. There are physical trainers, gyms galore, and even gadgets you can wear to help you maintain your physical well-being. While there may not be spiritual gadgets yet, there are therapists, religious leaders, friends, and family to help you maintain your spiritual spoke.

The mental spoke, though, is quite a bit more challenging. How can you tell if your brain is not as fit as it should be? You can't look at your brain in the mirror, and if it has a chemical or physical problem, the symptoms can take time to appear and might be mistaken for something else. There are tests we can take that are supposed to tell us how well our brains are doing, such as IQ tests. You can use these tests as a ruler to compare how you are doing as you age, but you shouldn't use them to compare yourself to someone else. For example, a person who scores 145 on an IQ test may not have a healthier mind than someone who scores 110. These tests should only be used to help you spot areas for improvement. Treating your mind as you would your physical body, by giving it regular and varied exercise, is the best thing you can do to prolong its health.

The rest of this chapter will focus on specific things you can do to keep your mental faculties honed throughout your life. No longer do you have to be tied to the belief that the brain simply shrinks and becomes less functional as we age. There are things you can do to stave off this atrophy and keep your mind sharp (barring disease and accidents) throughout your life.

Brain Usage

You have probably heard the adage that we only use ten percent of our brains. This is definitely not true. We use most of our brain, but at any given time we are using only parts of it. This is mainly due to how our brain is compartmentalized. The part of your brain that interprets what you hear is not the same part that controls where you walk or what you see. The brain is interconnected, but each area has its own set of responsibilities. There is a part that deals with languages, one for reasoning, and so on.

In order for you to maintain proper mental health, you need to exercise your whole brain. This will keep the neurons in each of its specific areas from atrophying. It is difficult to say just how much activity you need to keep your brain functioning at healthy levels, but doing a variety of activities can go a long way toward this goal. You cannot simply sit at a desk and expect your brain to get a full workout. The brain also gets exercise when you exercise your body. It is responsible for moving your limbs, keeping you from falling over, and a whole host of other activities you are unaware of.

In fact, you are oblivious to most of the activity going on in your head. If you had to think every time you did something, you would not be able to leave your house. There is just too much going on. The brain only brings to the foreground those things that you need to make decisions on or that represent some new information. For example, when you are learning something new, it is difficult and you have to stop and figure out what to do. Once you have mastered this new skill (such as riding a bike or juggling), the brain can push it to the background and concentrate on other things.

It is this "learning" that causes new connections to be made and growth to occur. The brain is constantly building new connections and making others go away. That is how neural pathways get established. The more these pathways get used, the stronger their connections become. This is both good and bad. It is good in that we can learn to do things really well without having to put much thought into it, but it is bad in that it makes change harder. People are creatures of habit because of this very trait. If it is a good habit it helps us, but if it is a bad habit it becomes difficult to undo.

And even good habits can have their downsides if we are trying to learn a new way of doing the same thing. For example, if my keyboard were to change, it would take me a long time to figure out the new layout and I would constantly try to type the old way. Figuring out new ways to do things will help keep your brain flexible and ready to adapt to an ever-changing world. We often hear about older people being "set" in their ways. This is because they have been doing the same things the same way for so long that their neural pathways are physically set and it takes a conscious effort to break out of these set ways. It is paramount that you keep your brain flexible and always keep trying new things. It will keep your brain, and therefore you, young.

Brain Health

Your brain needs nutrients just like the rest of your body and starts to suffer quickly if it doesn't get them. For example, if blood is cut off to the brain you will lose consciousness in about ten seconds. Ten seconds is a very short time, but you can recover fairly quickly if the blood flow returns. If the brain does not receive oxygen, the cells in the brain will start to die in as little as four minutes. The damage quickly becomes irreversible and can lead to death.

Recovery from lack of oxygen depends on the type of treatment, the environment (the colder the person is, the longer they can survive) and the individual. Complete lack of oxygen is obviously bad, but decreased amounts of oxygen can also be bad, such as in an environment full of smoke or smog. This oxygen-poor environment can lead to a poorly functioning brain and potentially cell death. Ideally, you should try to be in an environment that has adequate oxygen, surrounded by oxygen-producing organisms such as trees, grass and flowers. Oxygen is the primary requirement, but just one of many, for the brain to function optimally.

The brain needs the same vitamins and minerals as the rest of the body, but some nutrients are more important to brain health than others. The three I recommend most highly are Omega-3 fatty acids and the B complex of vitamins, with particular emphasis on folic acid. Omega-3 fatty acids are fats, and while this may seem counterintuitive at first, they are essential for your brain's overall health. They may also have many other brain benefits such as helping to combat depression.

The best way to obtain significant levels of Omega-3's is from cold-water fish such as cod, halibut and fresh tuna. There are other foods rich in Omega-3's such as eggs, but this is covered more in the fats section of the book. Folic acid is found in leafy vegetables such as spinach, beans of almost any sort, and citrus. If you eat meat, you can also get very high amounts from eating liver. The other B vitamins also occur in these foods at varying levels, but a well-rounded diet should get you an adequate amount.

Blood-Brain Barrier

This topic has more to do with preventing damage to your brain, but an understanding of the blood-brain barrier can also help you maintain its health. The brain is encapsulated by a barrier that keep the blood that circulates throughout your body separated from the fluid that surrounds the brain. The barrier lets in some things such as glucose for fuel, amino acids, oxygen, and other nutrients that it needs.

The blood-brain barrier is extremely effective at keeping bacteria out of the brain, which is why brain infections are so rare. It is also effective at keeping out antibodies, which makes it very hard for your body to fight off a brain infection if you do get one. Few antibiotics can cross the blood-brain barrier, which is probably a good thing for most infections, since you do not want anything in the brain that should not be there.

The important thing for your blood-brain barrier is to keep it intact. This means avoiding trauma to the head and excessive radiation and trying to keep infections to a minimum. It is also important to stay hydrated. Excessive concentrations of particles (like salt) can cause pressure to be exerted on the barrier, making it weak. You can also put pressure on it by taking too much medication or too many vitamins.

Your body has done a great job of putting up a protective barrier around your most precious organ, but it cannot keep you from trying to destroy it. There are many types of drugs (alcohol, THC, and barbiturates for example) that can cross through the barrier and do damage. You should minimize consumption of substances that cross the barrier. Even if you are taking these drugs for medical reasons, the less you can take, the better your brain will fare in the long run. Your body does not spend a lot of time and energy creating things it does not need, so keep that in mind and do some research on the medications you are putting into your body.

Feng Shui

To many people not familiar with feng shui, it might be hard to understand how this art could help with your mental well-being. Feng shui is the art of making spaces flow better. A very simple example is moving a chair so you do not have to walk around it to get to the kitchen. You may have walked around that chair so many times that you don't even think about it anymore, but your brain still has to account for it and that causes clutter in your brain. This clutter can make you tired, irritable, and less able to accomplish other tasks. This one item is probably not enough to worry about, but if your life is full of such clutter and obstacles, it is worth the time and effort to streamline your life.

When it comes to your brain, the little things matter. Take a stain on your carpet, for example. It may stay there for months or even years, and you consider it unimportant. Your brain, however, makes a note to ignore that spot so that it doesn't have to pay attention to it. This mental instruction takes up space and requires other thoughts to go around it. Ever notice how much better you feel after a room is cleaned? You might even feel like a weight has been lifted off your shoulders. This doesn't mean you have to become an obsessive cleaner, but it does mean you should take time to clean that carpet or remove whatever blights you come across during your daily life.

Feng shui is a topic unto itself and involves more than just making your small piece of the world flow better. There are spiritual aspects too, involved with more subtle features like art and lighting. These features can affect your mental and spiritual aspects, and eventually your physical as well. Making the effort to learn more about feng shui principles and apply them throughout your life is worthwhile. For the purposes of this book, we can focus on a few things to get you started.

- Reduce the clutter. If you don't need it, get rid of it (or at least get it out of sight).

- Move your furniture to make it easier to get from one room to the other and to get to the things you need most often.
- Ensure you have adequate, soft light where needed.

If you just follow these three steps, you are on your way to helping your mind function more efficiently and feeling better all around.

Exercise: Identify Your Paths Of Flow

In this exercise, you will probably need a fresh set of eyes. Preferably someone you trust but who does not spend a lot of time in your house (once you get past the morning part of the exercise anyway). You can also do this yourself, but try to pretend you are seeing your environment for the first time. The goal is to reduce the visual clutter and increase the flow of your environment with some simple steps. You will not have to knock down walls or do any sort of major repairs. We will just focus on what you can do with a minimal amount of effort to start getting the benefits of a more fluid living space. To complete this exercise, pick a day and start performing the steps below first thing in the morning.

1. When you wake up in the morning, take a moment before you get out of bed. Notice if you are comfortable and ask yourself these questions. Are you too hot or too cold? Do your bed and pillow provide the correct support for your body? Is the light too bright?
2. As you get up, notice if there is anything you have to maneuver around to go where you wish first thing in the morning. For example, do you have to make several turns to get out of the room or make an effort not to bump into items such as a bedpost, laundry basket or nightstand? You should have a relatively clear path out of your sleeping area as you give yourself time to awaken and begin your day.

3. While doing your morning routine, you should make a note of any difficulties that you encounter, such as having to search for a brush or fumble around to find your toothbrush. Is the bathroom area filled with items that you do not need in the morning? Excess clutter can be distracting even if you are not conscious of it.

4. As you prepare your breakfast and get dressed, mark how many trips you need to take to accomplish these tasks. For example, if you are a coffee and toast kind of person, you might want to keep the coffee maker, toaster, and coffee all in one location rather than on opposite sides of the kitchen. The same goes with getting dressed. Keeping your clothes organized will help you start your day on the right track. Better yet, on each night you could plan what you will wear the next day and have your clothes ready.

5. On your way to work or wherever you are going that day, think about the route you are taking and ask yourself if there might be a better way, perhaps leaving at a different time or taking an alternate route. A route that is pleasing to the eye or involves less hectic traffic might make your day happier even if it takes a bit longer to arrive.

6. Continue your day, asking yourself similar questions to those you began your morning with. Are there more pleasant ways to get to the places you need to go (like going past a fountain instead of through a sterile looking corridor)? Is the environment you are spending your day in comfortable and ergonomic? You should spend your day in an environment that helps you accomplish your tasks rather than one that makes you work around objects and circumstances to get things done.

Keeping It Fresh

Your brain was designed to conserve energy as a survival technique. Your ancestors did not have access to virtually unlimited calories and therefore had to make do with what they had. So there is no way around it – your brain doesn't want to work any harder than it has to. On top of that, your brain already consumes 25 percent of your calories in its normal functions, so it will resist doing extra work. You aren't lazy; you are just doing what nature has groomed you to do.

But conserving energy doesn't keep your brain fresh and growing. That will take effort on your part. You will have to push your brain beyond what nature intended. If you want your brain cells to replace themselves and perhaps even grow beyond what society has told us to expect, you will need to push your mind. Just as you push your body so your muscles will grow, you will have to exercise your brain. It doesn't matter how old you feel or how hard it might seem. You can make your brain create new connections and grow new cells.

The idea that your brain has to shrink as you enter your advanced years is only a myth. Statistics reflect this shrinkage because most people simply stop using their brains. Evolution hasn't given us a reason to keep using our brains beyond the requirements of producing offspring. Therefore, it has deemed that we do not need to keep feeding the brain and giving it valuable calories that could be used elsewhere or given to others who could further the evolutionary line. You have to remember that everything up to this point has been optimized to either produce offspring or to conserve energy. Making your brain last into your later years of life was not on that list.

Therefore you will have to fight nature to keep your brain fresh, but it is definitely within your grasp to do. You just have to want it bad enough and do what it takes to keep going. It is too easy to let things slide as most people do. Stay focused and keep track of your progress. That is the best way to keep your brain exercised so it will continue to serve you well throughout your life.

Male And Female Brains

A whole host of studies have been done on the differences between the male and female brain. One of these studies found that the male brain tends to act in a linear fashion and that females are better at multitasking. As far as the physical attributes of the brain are concerned, there do seem to be some differences. Knowing this, you could focus your tasks on the areas in which you are weaker. For example, I am a "typical" male and have trouble with multitasking, so I should focus on activities that improve those abilities. This approach should give your brain the best workout. Whenever something seems hard to figure out, it generally means you are pushing your brain, just like exercising your muscles. If you want your brain to grow, you will have to work it out.

The differences in brain structure start while still inside the womb. Differing levels of hormones cause the brain to develop in slightly different ways. This seems to continue to hold true later in life as well. One of these structural differences is the connection between the left and the right side of the brain, which is generally much stronger and thicker in females than in males. This means that women tend to be able to use both sides of their brains at the same time (hence the increased multitasking ability). There are some other differences in the way the brain is compartmentalized, the percentages of different types of cells and overall weight of the brain. (Weight has not been correlated with intelligence, however, so a bigger brain does not mean you are smarter.)

It is important to note that these differences are generalities and each person will have a unique brain architecture. This architecture is not fixed, though. It is just the base on which you can build. Your experiences throughout your life will shape your brain, as it changes throughout the day. Even when you sleep, you are making changes in the structure of your brain. You are constantly strengthening some pathways while others atrophy.

You should take time to identify those areas you are strong in (like multitasking, language skills, or spatial orientation) and those you need to spend time on to improve.

CHAPTER 5: ACTIVITIES FOR A BETTER YOU

Biking

Mental: 20%
Physical: 50%
Spiritual: 20%

Riding your bike can be great for you and for the environment. It is good for your legs and gentle on your joints. If you use it to get to work or to run errands, you will have the extra benefit of helping out the environment. Not everyone can ride their bike everywhere they need to go, but every time you can, you reduce the amount of carbon dioxide going into the air. There is also a spiritual element in that you get to enjoy the world around you on a more personal level than you would in a car.

Mountain biking is an even more intense version of biking. It is great exercise and can truly push your limits, but it can also cause you some serious bodily harm. Almost everyone I know who mountain bikes has broken some bones or been seriously hurt. This undermines the benefits of mountain biking. Therefore, my recommendation is to do mountain biking with safety in mind. It is great for your body, mind, and spirit as long as you do it safely.

Board Games

Mental: 50%
Physical: 10%
Spiritual: 50%

In the age of smartphones and tablets, you might not think board games would still be relevant, but they remain a great way to work your brain as well as interact with your friends and family. There are few other activities that can match the interaction of playing board games. They promote teamwork and exercise your brain, two very positive influences today's culture should promote and that digital technology cannot replace. I am also including group activities like charades in this category. Any game that brings a group together and involves working your brain counts as a board game.

Boating

Mental: 33%
Physical: 50%
Spiritual: 33%

For our purposes, boating refers to kayaking or canoeing in a natural environment, although other types of boating have benefits too. Boating provides excellent exercise for your arms and back but doesn't do much for your legs unless you carry your boat a significant distance. It also exercises your mind because you have to look ahead and do route planning based on your environment. You notice your surroundings more intently than you normally would, and during the leisurely parts of your trip you can sit back and soak in the beauty of Mother Nature.

The additional benefits of boating have to do with the element of water. Being on the water is good for your spirit, and since you should not be boating alone, you have the added benefit of connecting with others. Moving water generates negative ions that elevate your mood and bring a sense of well-being. The sounds of rushing water are beneficial too, especially if you are stressed or depressed. These sounds can lower your blood pressure and bring a sense of calm. Being on the water is not purely beneficial, though. It also introduces an element of danger. People die boating even in the calmest of waters, so you should never go boating alone under any circumstances. Even the best boater can have an off day and need the help of friends.

Bowling

Mental: 33%
Physical: 33%
Spiritual: 33%

While not as popular as it used to be, bowling is still a great way to get some exercise and see some of your friends, as long as you don't consume too many of the terrible food options at most bowling alleys. Becoming competent at bowling does take some effort. It can improve your hand-eye coordination and give you a decent leg workout if you are trying to bowl correctly. When I have not gone bowling in a while, I can definitely feel it in my legs the next day. In any case, it is a good excuse to go hang out with friends and almost anybody can do it, even people in wheelchairs. It beats sitting at a bar and trying to have a conversation over loud music.

Now that computer games have gotten more sophisticated, you can "bowl" at home on your video hardware. This does not equate to going out and actually bowling. There are some of the same spiritual benefits if you do this activity with your friends, but not nearly as many of the physical and mental benefits as actual bowling provides. Of course, it's better than doing nothing, especially if you go through the motions as if you were at the bowling alley.

Cardio

Mental: 20%
Physical: 66%
Spiritual: 20%

Cardio is anything that gets you to an elevated heart rate. For this particular grouping, you can consider it anything that you do on an elliptical or treadmill machine. Generally, this does not involve your mental or spiritual spokes much, but you can multitask and do other things while you do cardio (for example you could practice a new language). On the plus side, it is great for your heart, helps keep your bones strong, increases your metabolism, and burns a considerable number of calories. Another benefit is that most cardio activities are fairly low-impact, so they minimize wear and tear on your joints. Many of us are often confined to an indoor activity, and this is one you should include in your regimen if you cannot reach an elevated heart rate at least three times a week in other ways. You should maintain this elevated heart rate for at least twenty minutes, so plan on thirty minutes of cardio to give yourself five minutes on each side to warm up and cool down.

There are lots of different types of equipment on the market to help increase your cardiovascular health. This can make it very convenient if you have space where you live, but it is also worthwhile to visit your local gym so you can use a variety of machines and be part of your community. This can increase the spiritual component of this activity greatly. Also, you can get to know your neighbors and form a more cohesive community.

Crosswords

Mental: 50%
Physical: 10%
Spiritual: 33% (50% if done with another person)

Crossword puzzles are an excellent way to keep your mind sharp. With their help you can learn new words and aspects of culture you don't normally come across and build problem-solving skills. Crosswords come in a variety of types and difficulties, so some are bound to be perfect for you. You can start with the easier ones and work your way up to the really hard ones. Just increasing your knowledge can bring you a certain satisfaction and give you a general sense of well-being. Working with another person can bring you closer to that person and increase your team-building skills. Solving crosswords is also one of the cheapest activities you can do. Most newspapers have a daily crossword in them, there are tons of crosswords online, and almost all the magazines in airplanes have them.

One of the best benefits of crossword puzzles is that they can actually change the way you think about solving problems. Many of us get stuck thinking there is one right answer to a problem and if that answer doesn't work, we give up. As we become older, this inability to think of other solutions (or "think outside the box") is far too common. Crossword puzzles show us that even if a problem seems impossible at first, if we attack it from different angles we can eventually solve it. Every older person I have met who works crossword puzzles regularly has been sharp-witted and a quick thinker. I hope to be one of those sharp-witted older people one day and still doing crossword puzzles regularly.

Dancing

Mental: 33%
Physical: 66%
Spiritual: 33%

Dancing is great exercise as well as a way to connect with others. Even dancing by yourself can benefit all aspects of your being tremendously. The type of dancing can vary the benefit greatly, so you can take the percentages listed above as a minimum. No matter what kind of dancing you do, you will benefit from moving your body to music so your mind and muscles develop neuronal connections. Dancing with others also benefits your spiritual side. You can develop community connections and deeper interpersonal connections with other people in the process, strengthening both your spiritual spoke and the spiritual spokes of others.

Languages

Mental: 100%
Physical: 20%
Spiritual: 50%

Learning a new language is a difficult task, and becoming fluent is even harder (something I have yet to do so far). It is one of the most difficult things your brain can do and therefore one of the best exercises for it. Even if you never become fluent, just knowing some words of another language works your brain and keeps it pliable. And by studying a culture's language you can learn a lot about that culture that would be inaccessible to you otherwise. Each language reflects the mindset of the culture that uses it and can be a unique window into that culture.

Hiking

Mental: 33%
Physical: 50%
Spiritual: 33%

Hiking is a wonderful way to get some great exercise and expand your mind and spirit at the same time. There is a great deal of difference in the hikes that are available in the world. Some are truly life-changing experiences such as hiking up Mount Fuji or the Tongariro crossing in New Zealand. Those hikes will stay with you for the rest of your life. But even less momentous hikes are still quite beneficial. To get the most out of a hike, you should combine a physical challenge with varying terrain. The brain has to do a tremendous amount of work to properly coordinate your leg movements while maintaining your balance. The visual stimuli also work out the brain as well as the eyes. Combine that with a loaded backpack and you have a workout that really challenges your legs, improves your posture, and increases your bone density, helping prevent osteoporosis. If you live in a very dense area it might be hard to get to a place where you can do a proper hike, but if you use your imagination you can do some urban hiking in most cities.

Housework

Mental: 20%
Physical: 50%
Spiritual: 33%

Most of us think of housework as something to be avoided rather than an activity that can keep us healthy. Doing housework yourself rather than hiring somebody to do it has many benefits. Vacuuming or sweeping can be a great workout for your abs, your arms, and your back. Plus it can help you burn calories if you are trying to lose those few extra pounds. A clean house will help you be more organized and provide an enjoyable environment in which to live. It makes the air around you easier to breathe, increasing your oxygen intake and making allergic reactions less likely.

There is a spiritual component to keeping your surroundings clean and tidy as well. Being clean and organized will make you feel better about your life. It has been shown that a dirty neighborhood is more likely to have an increase in crime, especially vandalism and theft. A clean environment lets people know that the area is cared for, so they are less apt to damage it. It is the same way with your house. If someone comes in and sees a house well taken care of, they are less likely to dirty it up.

Isometrics

Mental: 33%
Physical: 33%
Spiritual: 0%

I have spent much of my life sitting at a desk and discovered isometrics as a way to maintain muscle tone without having to do much movement. In case you don't know, isometrics is the act of contracting your muscles without moving. You can think of it as flexing in place. In order for this activity to count you should do it periodically throughout the day. Each time doesn't have to take very long. You don't want to cramp up as you do it. Doing isometrics can help maintain your posture as well as counterbalance the detrimental effects of sitting at a desk. It will not replace other types of exercise but it is a valuable addition to your regimen of maintaining your physical well-being. Isometrics work your mental spoke too because of the significant mental energy and concentration required to properly perform these exercises. They do get easier as you get more practice, though.

Martial Arts

Mental: 33%
Physical: 100%
Spiritual: 50%

Martial arts is a practice I have a lot of mixed opinions about. Under the right circumstances it can strengthen your wheel in ways few other activities can match. However, under the wrong circumstances it can cause great damage to your spiritual and physical well-being. When starting a practice you can generally get a feel for how the training will proceed. The keys are to avoid getting physically injured and to focus on the protection of yourself and those around you. If you and your instructor keep those two goals in mind, your practice can achieve quite lofty goals of spiritual and physical fulfillment.

It is also a great way to stay mentally sharp, as there is a lot to memorize and the hand- (and foot-)eye coordination required really make your brain work. Overall, it is definitely worth pursuing and can yield lifelong benefits that go far beyond self-defense.

Memory Games

Mental: 66%
Physical: 0%
Spiritual: 0%

Memory games focus on a single component of your brain but are still important. We focus on this component in school when we have to memorize facts and how to spell words. Unfortunately, once we leave school we have little incentive to keep this part of the brain active. We now have smartphones and computers to remember all the little details of our lives for us. I am guilty of this too. I only know a few phone numbers of the people I care about, and if I lost my phone I wouldn't be able to call them until I got a new phone and had my contacts restored. This fact indicates that I have let one of my major mental muscles become flabby.

The part of our brain responsible for memorizing items is one of the most important parts. If you let it decay from disuse, you are seriously compromising your mental spoke, which could ruin your entire wheel. You can see concrete examples of this decline in people who have Alzheimer's disease. Having a good memory is not proof against such diseases, but allowing your memory to degrade can bring about similar results.

Memory games and memorizing the important facts in your life can help you stave off this decay and actually increase your capacity to memorize items. There are simple online games you can play, or you can use cards to find matches. Another thing you can do is memorize the important phone numbers in your life and maybe even the addresses of those you care about. Whatever you do, remember that working on your memory is important.

Playing Cards

Mental: 33%
Physical: 10%
Spiritual: 50%

Here I do not mean gambling, but sitting around with a bunch of friends and playing a game like gin rummy. Playing cards can help with math skills as well as other cognitive functions, depending on the type of game you are playing. There are whole hosts of games to choose from, and with more coming on the market all the time. The best thing about playing cards is that it gives you a chance to connect with your friends and family, allowing for face-to-face interaction that you cannot get by watching television. You can really get to know somebody just by playing an evening of cards with them. This can help achieve a sense of community and happiness too as long as you don't get too serious about who wins and who loses. Even if your opponents overly celebrate, you can still enjoy the socializing and realize in the end it is just a game. The only pitfall with playing cards is the tendency to overindulge. It is easy to sit there and stuff your face with fattening food and soda or alcohol. While food and drink can make playing cards more enjoyable, it only takes a little planning to make the event a healthy and tasty one.

Reading

Mental: 66%
Physical: 20%
Spiritual: 33%

I firmly believe you should read something every day, even if it is the back of a cereal box. Ideally, you should read a wide variety of materials to get the full mental benefit, but any sort of reading is beneficial. It is also a workout for your eyes. You also need to balance eye workouts by focusing on objects far away, but reading gives your eyes a good close-up workout. Reading can take you around the world and open your mind to a multitude of experiences without ever leaving your home. Technology has made millions of books available to people everywhere. Many of these books are even free to download. Despite the ease and portability of e-readers, I still prefer to have a good old-fashioned paper book to read. Whatever way you prefer to read, the important thing is that you try to do it every day that you can.

Roller Skating

Mental: 33%
Physical: 66%
Spiritual: 33%

Roller skating is experiencing a resurgence lately, especially in the form of roller derby. It's a great way to exercise your legs and meet up with your friends. It requires considerable coordination between your muscles and your brain, hence the benefits to your mental spoke. Roller skating is a bit intimidating if you have never done it before, but with a little practice you will soon be circling the rink with the best of them. The only concern is avoiding injuries. It is a low-contact activity normally, but accidents do happen. You can mitigate this danger by wearing appropriate safety gear, especially if you are participating in a roller derby function.

Role-Playing Games

Mental: 66%
Physical: 20%
Spiritual: 66%

I am talking about your old dice-and-paper role-playing here, but some of the same benefits can be found using the computer. There is something about immersing yourself into another character that stretches your mind and rewards your spirit. Interacting with others in a cooperative way can benefit you in many aspects of your life. The only danger is eating too many snacks and sodas, which would make your gaming a net negative rather than a healthy activity. If you can avoid weight gain, role-playing is one of the best activities for expanding your mind. You have to think outside the box to solve the truly hard problems. Plus you have a creative outlet to develop a unique character that lets you explore parts of your life that you may find difficult to do otherwise. It also creates a safe environment to meet other people and form lasting bonds that can strengthen your spiritual spoke.

Running

Mental: 33%
Physical: 80%
Spiritual: 33%

Personally, I have never been a big fan of running, but it is a great way to keep your lower body and heart in shape. It doesn't do much for your upper body, but it gets your heart rate up much better than walking does. I don't do much running because I try to protect my knees. Running, especially on pavement or concrete, can put a lot of pressure on your joints. But you can also get a certain amount of spiritual fulfillment from running. It will challenge you and allow you to set goals you can reach for. Achieving these goals will increase your confidence in other areas of your life as well. The mental benefit comes from the enormous number of calculations your brain undertakes to keep you moving forward without falling over. This benefit is intensified when the course covers varied terrain, as in trail running. Softer ground is also easier on your joints as long as you do not trip over obstacles and injure yourself.

Singing

Mental: 50%
Physical: 33%
Spiritual: 66%

Singing is something anyone can do. Even if you don't think you can sing well you can do it at home, especially with the recent proliferation of karaoke machines and video games that involve singing. Your vocal cords are muscles and need to be exercised just like all muscles. Music really reaches down into your inner being and lets you express yourself in ways that can greatly benefit your spiritual self. Additionally, you can add singing to many other life activities. You can sing while you clean your house or in the shower or just whenever you feel the need to sing. Everyone should sing sometimes, but many of us are self-conscious about how we sound. If this is the case for you, find a place where you can sing in privacy until you feel comfortable letting others hear your singing voice. There is even greater benefit in singing with others, as you can develop a sense of belonging and community that is hard to achieve with other activities. Finally, it works a specific part of your mind that can help you in many other seemingly unrelated areas such as math. And if you can't sing out loud, you can always sing in your head.

Sudoku

Mental: 66%
Physical: 10%
Spiritual: 20%

The brain needs many different types of exercise and math is one area where most of us fail to get enough. Sudoku is one of the few mental math exercises that can be found easily and is quite enjoyable to many. You can start off with the easy ones and work your way up as you get better. Even if you just stick with the easy ones, though, it is still working a new part of your brain, encouraging growth and connections. Luckily, Sudoku has become very popular over the last few years and can be found in newspapers, in magazines, and online. All you have to do is find some Sudoku puzzles and get to it. At first, the puzzles might seem quite difficult, but give yourself some time and try to be patient. After you successfully finish a few of them, you may even find that you enjoy them.

Surfing

Mental: 50%
Physical: 100%
Spiritual: 50%

I will admit that I have never done much real surfing on a board. However, I have done a lot of body surfing and boogie boarding, and while those are not exactly the same, the benefits are similar. Being on the water and experiencing the rush of the wave are life-changing. Nothing can replace catching that wave just right and having it hurtle you through space and time. You become one with nature and ride it for all it is worth. It takes a special blend of mental, physical, and spiritual strength to make that happen. It is one of the best exercises you can do for your wheel, and you will not regret doing it.

It is not easy for everyone to get to a surfing spot. Only a lucky few have the opportunity to surf regularly. The number of surfing spots in the world is pretty small but growing constantly thanks to wetsuits and people willing to challenge society's norms. There are many artificial waves that are popping up across the world too. These may not provide as much benefit, but they are still a great way to get some exercise and experience many of the same benefits that surfing in nature brings. Plus you can get some practice so when you do get the chance to go surfing in the wild, your skills will be honed.

Swimming

Mental: 20%

Physical: 75%
Spiritual: 20%

Few exercises work out the entire body as well as swimming. It works the arms, back, legs, and core as well as the lungs and heart. I am primarily talking about swimming laps, but swimming in a lake or ocean can do the same thing. Any time in the water is generally a good thing. It doesn't matter much what kind of water you are in, since your body mainly focuses on the repetitive motions swimming requires. You get into a zone that you lets you concentrate on working out, not worrying about your surroundings. It truly is one of the best exercises to strengthen your physical spoke. There is a small mental benefit, but once the rhythm has been achieved, not much brain activity is needed. The spiritual aspect is pretty low too because of the lack of interaction with your surroundings. Swimming takes considerable physical effort and leaves little room for other parts of the wheel. Even with the predominant focus on the physical spoke, it is still great exercise.

Tennis

Mental: 33%
Physical: 66%
Spiritual: 33%

Competitive sports are great for staying in physical shape and have spiritual and mental benefits as well. The downside is that many of these sports are fraught with injuries that can sideline you for months, if not years. Tennis provides many of the benefits of other sports such as football or soccer, but the likelihood of a serious injury is much lower. Injuries tend to be cumulative and can greatly affect the quality of your later life. Tennis is great for your cardiovascular health and hand-eye coordination and strengthens your legs as well as your arms.

Another benefit of playing tennis is that you can both cooperate and compete with your friends and meet new people in the process. It is also a fairly low-cost way to exercise. Once you buy the racket and a few balls, you can find free courts in many communities. Tennis rises and falls in popularity but has enough devotees that you can usually find a number of courts near you with a little searching.

Travel

Mental: 50%
Physical: 20%
Spiritual: 50%

When I put travel down as an activity, I was thinking of travel to a place you have never been. This kind of travel really opens up your mind and can do wonders for your spirit. Your brain wakes up to your new surroundings, taking in all of this new information, and creates a multitude of new connections and memories. Your normal day-to-day life can blend together after a while and seem like one big blur, but when you travel every day is filled with new and memorable moments. Not every day of travel will be enjoyable, but every day will have its share of adventures that can help you grow and strengthen your wheel.

When you do travel, it helps to take pictures of the people and environments you encounter (buildings, beaches, mountains, etc.) so that you can look at them later and spur memories, exciting the neurons in your brain to form and strengthen connections. Another great way to bring back these memories is to keep a journal you can refer to in the future or to find that special souvenir that really embodies the place you visited. If you do find a location that holds a special place in your heart, try to keep something that reminds you of that spot where you can see it every day and remember what made it so special to you.

Walking

Mental: 33%

Physical: 50%
Spiritual: 33%

Walking is truly one of the simple pleasures in life that has a multitude of benefits. It helps keep your bones strong, works out your legs and heart, and allows you to truly enjoy the surroundings you pass through. Varying your path will also increase both the mental and spiritual aspects of your walking. Walking the same path every day makes the brain notice less and less of the path that you take. You can also increase the mental and physical challenge by choosing a path with varied terrain. Your brain and muscles then have to work together to determine where to place your feet rather than just proceeding on "automatic." Choosing a path with natural beauty will increase the enjoyment of the walk and thus the spiritual benefit you receive.

Too, you can learn more about your neighborhood and the people in it by walking in the area where you live. Far too often we live next to people for years without ever getting to know them. Walking lets you become closer to your neighbors and increases your sense of community. In times of crisis you will have to depend on your neighbors, so it is best to know them in advance.

Writing

Mental: 100%
Physical: 20%
Spiritual: 100%

Writing is the gateway to the inner you. Even if you never publish a single thing, it is important for you to put to paper (or to the internet cloud) the things that are important to you. When you write, it is a window into the inner you and allows you to express yourself in a safe environment. The act of putting your feelings down lets you explore them and work through them in a way you could not otherwise.

Many of us (myself included) would like to be able to produce a written work good enough to be enjoyed by more than just ourselves. Be warned that though this task has its own benefits, it is a much more involved ordeal and can take years to accomplish. Writing a full-length book requires dedication, time, and other resources. I commend your efforts if you do set yourself on this path, and I can only hope that you are able to achieve the enjoyment of completing a novel. There is nothing like being able to hold your book in your own hands and know that you were the one who brought it into being.

Weight Lifting

Mental: 20%
Physical: 75%
Spiritual: 20%

People tend to lift weights either all the time or not at all. Doing some sort of resistance-type exercise is essential for maintaining bone density, crucial to prevent bone damage later in life, and should be part of everyone's lifestyle. Lifting weights is a great way to get the benefits of resistance exercise in a short time. It also builds muscle and increases metabolism.

There are a lot of different ways to lift weights, and if you are just starting out you should work with a personal trainer or someone who knows what they are doing. It is easy to hurt yourself lifting weights if you are not knowledgeable enough. One wrong lift can sideline you for weeks or even months. This is not to scare you off, as weight lifting is a great way to strengthen your physical spoke. My advice would be to start off slow and give yourself time to heal between sessions. If you want to lift weights more often, you can switch between different body groups (i.e., do upper body one day and legs the next).

Video Games

Mental: 40%
Physical: 20%

Spiritual: 20%

Video games can be a valid activity to help improve the spokes of your wheel. This is one activity where the benefits actually diminish as you do more. You should minimize the amount of time that you spend video gaming, although the benefits vary greatly depending on the kind of game. Many of the newer video games include a significant amount of physical activity and spending time with others. If you do play a lot of video games, try to include a mix of different games so you can maximize benefit for all three of your spokes. But no matter how varied your video games are, it is still important to get away from the computer or television often enough. Also, be careful of sitting in the same spot for hours on end. This can cause a whole host of physical issues from muscle atrophy to spinal curvature. There is nothing wrong with video games. Just remember that there is much, much more to life.

Yard Work

Mental: 33%
Physical: 66%
Spiritual: 33%

If you are lucky enough to have a yard, you should take the opportunity to get out and take care of it rather than hiring somebody else. People will pay money to go to the gym when they could get the same workout in their yard. Raking leaves is great for your back and your core. Mowing the grass can be just as good as spending time on an elliptical machine. Yard work is also an excellent way to commune with nature and connect with your surroundings. Many of us have allergies that prevent us from doing some yard work tasks at certain times of year, but there are still lots of other tasks to choose from.

You can get additional benefits from helping neighbors who cannot do their own yard work or who just need a hand to speed it up. You will feel better inside and look better outside, plus you will be helping maintain the quality of your neighborhood. Also, you might need a hand with some tasks in the future, and it is a lot easier and cheaper to ask a friend or neighbor to help.

Yoga

Mental: 33%
Physical: 100%
Spiritual: 100%

Few activities that you can perform are as fulfilling as yoga. It works the entire body and provides a spiritual outlet that is rare among physical activities. Once you consider the hand-eye coordination and the mental concentration it requires, yoga is probably the best activity you can add to your repertoire. If you only do one physical exercise, this would be your best choice. It combines strength, endurance, and flexibility, and it burns calories. There are two main types of yoga, referred to as yin yoga and yang yoga. In yin yoga the emphasis is on lengthening your muscles and holding stretching poses for longer periods of time. Yang yoga is more aerobic and can be thought of strengthening your muscles (including your heart), like more traditional exercises. I cannot recommend yoga highly enough. If you have never tried it, please go out and try it today. I was well into my thirties before I first encountered yoga and I have never looked back. I try to do it at least three times a week when I can and am never disappointed. Some yoga classes are better than others, but any yoga is better than no yoga. Below are some of the common types of yoga you can find in a studio near you. Luckily, most places are catching the yoga craze, and it's likely there is a place to practice yoga near you. Of course, you can always do yoga by yourself. All you need is about 20 square feet of flat space.

Bikram Yoga

A typical Bikram yoga class runs for 90 minutes and is the same set of 26 movements repeated over and over. The room is heated to about 105 degrees Fahrenheit (Bikram is often referred to as "hot yoga," but there are several different kinds of hot yoga), which causes you to sweat a lot during the class. If you are new to yoga, this type may be too intense to start off with. Just remember that during yoga you can always stop and rest. Don't overdo it. The only competition in yoga is with yourself. The nice thing about it is that you can expect the same class no matter where you go: Every Bikram class should be much the same. It is a guaranteed workout and a serious calorie burner. Plus, like most yoga classes, it works out the entire body.

Hatha Yoga

Traditionally hatha yoga could be used to mean any type of yoga, but today it usually refers to a gentle and relaxing form of yoga that does not use flow between the positions. If you are new to yoga, this is a good type to learn the basic poses so that you can expand upon them in future sessions. Even after you have taken yoga for years, hatha yoga is still an excellent way to ground yourself and find inner peace and harmony. Like all forms of yoga, it also helps with maintaining balance, flexibility, and general movement of parts of your body that may not get a chance to move during your normal daily routine. Hatha can be especially helpful for reducing stress, and it is very low-impact so can be helpful in recovering from injuries or after you have been sick.

Vinyasa Yoga

This type of yoga links breath with movement. It is generally a vigorous workout with yin yoga at the end of the class. Each vinyasa class is different, so getting a good instructor is very important. Generally, vinyasa yoga will leave you with the feeling that you have been worked out hard. The room is generally heated, but not as hot as for Bikram yoga. The room is kept warm to make the muscles more flexible and less likely to cramp up. It is often said that if you are mindfully breathing, then you are doing vinyasa yoga and everything else is just an extension. That is because the entire class is centered around your breath. You breathe in and you perform a movement. Then you breathe out and perform another movement. This is my favorite type of yoga because it varies from class to class and provides a very good all-over workout.

Yin Yoga

At first glance yin yoga may seem easier in that there is not a lot of movement, but it can be deceptively strenuous. The poses are held for several minutes each, which requires considerable flexibility and often endurance too. Of the different types of yoga, this one is the hardest for me because I find it very difficult to stay still. Additionally, many of the poses are physically hard to maintain, requiring considerable strength, especially in the core area. Yin yoga is designed to lengthen your muscles, increase your flexibility, and allow your mind to explore areas that may be troubling you. The longer you hold the pose, the more your mind can explore issues in your life that may be troubling you. This provides an excellent opportunity to tackle these issues and work through them. You should balance others types of yoga and physical exercise with yin yoga so that your muscles are given the chance to be fully stretched out. It is the one type of yoga I personally avoid but is probably the one I should do more often.

12 Weeks To A Better You

To help kick-start you, you can use the page after this section as a template to help you track your activities and encourage you to diversify the amount of energy you expend on each of your spokes. To start with, write down each activity you do and the points associated with each activity (for example 33% is equal to 33 points), then see how many points you have at the end of the week. At first I would aim for 300 points in each category per week so you have a goal to shoot towards. The act of measuring your progress will help you stay motivated and hopefully help you balance your wheel and strengthen each of your spokes. By the end of the twelve weeks you should have established a firm foundation for healthy habits that you will hopefully continue for many years. These habits you form will go a long way toward keeping the entire wheel of you healthy, happy, and youthful.

The chart only allows for a couple of activities per day, but you can write in more if you can do them or use another method to keep track, such as your phone or computer. In reality, for most of us who have a normal work week (and I do consider taking care of kids as working), two activities a day is quite a feat to accomplish, and you should be commended if you can accomplish that many regularly. You can probably do more on the weekends (if you are a normal worker bee), but it would be hard to do more than two a day on workdays. Between sleep, work, and eating, not much of the day is left to do activities for ourselves, which is why we have to optimize what little time we have to work with. I purposely did not put time limits on the activities. It is up to you to determine if you did enough for it to count. I personally count anything that approaches 30 minutes in length. You can adjust this based on the activity, how much effort you are putting into it, and how hard that particular task is for you. The idea of the points is to motivate you and give you a way to note your progress, not to stress you out.

Week 1

Day	Activity	Mental	Physical	Spiritual
Sunday	_____________	_______	_______	_______
	_____________	_______	_______	_______
Monday	_____________	_______	_______	_______
	_____________	_______	_______	_______
Tuesday	_____________	_______	_______	_______
	_____________	_______	_______	_______
Wednesday	_____________	_______	_______	_______
	_____________	_______	_______	_______
Thursday	_____________	_______	_______	_______
	_____________	_______	_______	_______
Friday	_____________	_______	_______	_______
	_____________	_______	_______	_______
Saturday	_____________	_______	_______	_______
	_____________	_______	_______	_______
Total Points		_______	_______	_______

Day	Activity	Mental	Physical	Spiritual
Sunday	Crossword	50	10	33
	Cardio	20	66	20
Monday	Off	_______	_______	_______
Tuesday	Walking	33	50	33
Wednesday	Vinyasa Yoga	33	100	100
Thursday	Swimming	20	75	20
	Cardio	50	10	20
Friday	Off	_______	_______	_______
Saturday	Singing	50	33	66
Total Points		256	344	292

AFTERWORD

There is a lot of information to digest in this book. If you have made it this far, you are well on your way. Don't try to push yourself too hard at first. Maintaining yourself is not a quick-fix project. It is an ongoing commitment to yourself that can give you a happier, healthier, and more fulfilling life. Take some time to ease into taking better care of the whole you. Start by removing those things that prevent your progress and prioritize yourself so you can be better for you and for those you care about. This process will probably require some major adjustments, but there are few obstacles you cannot overcome if you put your mind to it. I personally hope that you have a long and fruitful life and that you can make yourself and the world around you a little better each and every day. And if you do not achieve that goal today, try again tomorrow. Eventually it will become a habit and you won't even have to think about it. It will be as natural as breathing.

ABOUT THE AUTHOR

Michael Doyle

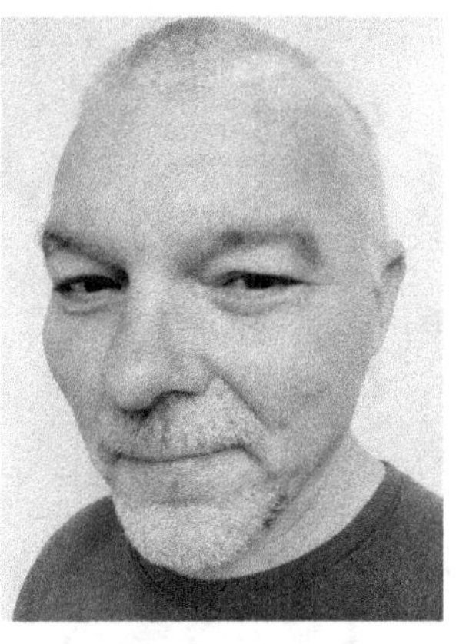

Michael Doyle has spent most of his life in the software field but has two degrees in biomedical engineering from Vanderbilt University, which helps explain his lifelong desire to understand how the human body works and how to keep it at a high level of functioning. He has lived in a variety of places across the United States and has been fortunate enough to have four wonderful children, all of whom have helped him grow and learn and, most of all, have given him the desire to be around for a long, long time so he can enjoy their company for many years to come. In his spare time he tries to enjoy the outdoors, whether at the beach or on a hike in the woods.